The Stroke Patient:
Principles of Rehabilitation

The Stroke Patient: Principles of Rehabilitation

MARGARET JOHNSTONE M.C.S.P.

Illustrated by Estrid Barton

Foreword by Professor Bernard Isaacs M.D. F.R.C.P.
Charles Hayward Professor of Geriatric Medicine,
University of Birmingham

CHURCHILL LIVINGSTONE
EDINBURGH LONDON AND NEW YORK 1976

CHURCHILL LIVINGSTONE

Medical Division of Longman Group Limited

Distributed in the United States of America by
Longman Inc., 19 West 44th Street, New
York,N.Y. 10036 and by associated
companies,
branches and representatives throughout
the world.

ISBN 0 443 01487 6

Library of Congress Cataloging in Publication Data

Johnstone, Margaret.
    The stroke patient.

    Includes index.
    1. Stroke patients—Rehabilitation. I. Title.
RC388.5.J62   616.8′1′06   76-16048

Printed in Hong Kong

Foreword

The human brain, in the complexity of its structure, in the range and richness of its function, represents the highest achievement of evolution; and endows Man with his unique mastery over space and time. Disease of the brain destroys this dominance. When the disease is sudden and massive the integrity of the personality is catastrophically disrupted. Such is the effect of stroke disease. The condition is even more poignant when it afflicts people, as often it does, at the height of their creative lives. It might be expected that every detail of treatment of the stroke patient would be deeply ingrained into medical students and doctors in training, to enable them to give the maximum help to the victims of this tragic disease. But it is not so. Standard text books of medicine, and even of neurology, have little to say on the subject. Medical examinations rarely include questions on the treatment of stroke. In the daily practice of many hospitals, with some notable exceptions, the work of stroke rehabilitation goes on largely without benefit of medical guidance. Why many doctors thus deprive themselves of participation in a medical activity which is scientifically fascinating and therapeutically rewarding remains a mystery. But with or without the collaboration of medical colleagues, physiotherapists, occupational therapists, speech therapists and nurses have observed the behaviour of stroke patients, and have worked out for themselves the best way of promoting recovery and minimising disability.

Margaret Johnstone is a physiotherapist who has thought deeply about the stroke patients under her care, and has arrived at the conclusion that stroke rehabilitation must be the work of a team in which every member is aware of the methods used by others. The patient thus receives a consistent and comprehensible scheme of management. The team includes everyone who comes in contact with the patient, and none more so than the professional and auxiliary nurses who are so intimately involved with lifting, turning and assisting the patient in the early dark days of disability. It is at this stage that the potential for good and for harm is at its greatest, and Mrs Johnstone rightly addresses much of her work to these vital deliverers of care. At a different level she has much to impart to her professional colleagues. Her methods are electric; but they are soundly based on neurophysiological principles. They have given her consistently good clinical results, and they make sense. She has set them down in order to communicate to others the principles which she has found to be important. Her writing is so direct that she seems to be speaking urgently through the pages; emphasising correct practices and warning against wrong ones. She has been fortunate in obtaining the services of an exceptionally gifted artist, her niece, Estrid Barton, to convey in meticulously clear line drawings precisely how it should be done.

The great need in stroke rehabilitation, as in the management of many other areas of disability, is not just for new knowledge but for the wider dissemination and application of existing knowledge. These needs are well met in Margaret Johnstone's book.

Birmingham, 1976   BERNARD ISAACS

Preface

In writing this book, step by step, I have realised that it is a work which began over thirty years ago when I first set foot in my physiotherapy training school, and it developed over the years as a result of the influence a few special people have had on my career. Most of them I met in the course of duty and all of them became respected and sincere friends. Accordingly, I would like to acknowledge the debt I owe to them and I would like them to know what their encouragement has meant to me.

I give my thanks and gratitude to:

Miss M.I.V. Mann, whose enthusiasm carried me hopefully through a wartime training and taught me that only the best is good enough.

Professor Norman Dott, sadly posthumously, who taught me all I know about re-education of balance in his wartime unit for gunshot wounds of the head, and who also taught me that a positive approach and a cheerful spirit are essential ingredients in any rehabilitation programme.

Mr W.V. Anderson, who encouraged me as a student and later, during seventeen years of caring for the disabled child, also taught me to set my sights high and never to accept the second-rate.

Miss M.D. Gardiner, who spent three weeks of intensive tutoring initiating me into the mysteries of Proprioceptive Neuromuscular Facilitation.

Dr David Seaton, who gave me a free hand while I worked with his stroke patients at Chalmers Hospital, Edinburgh, and encouraged me to spend six years finding an answer to the problem of the residual disability of the hemiplegic arm.

Elizabeth Neate, who made herself my right hand during those six years and became my indispensable assistant.

Aline Schofield, who taught me all I know about occupational therapy.

Jennifer Dunlop, who listened to my many questions with patience and led me towards a fuller understanding of speech and language disorder.

Victoria Hards, who shared my training days and who, during the last eighteen months, has encouraged me to write this book while I have seen what is being done for the elderly in her rather special unit at Liberton Hospital.

Estrid Barton, my niece, who has given her lively talent freely, producing diagrams that are self-explanatory while her twin brother likened the brain to a telephone exchange.

My son David, who, with unfailing good humour, posed repeatedly for the necessary photographs to help the artist.

This book is dedicated to all of you.

Edinburgh,   M.J.
1976

Contents

1. The Team

In recent years the stroke has come to be seen as one of the major health hazards of modern life. Almost every medical ward in our hospitals has a percentage of stroke, or hemiplegic, patients. All geriatric hospitals have a large proportion of hemiplegic victims among the inmates—and I use the word 'victim' deliberately. The number of these patients in Britain to-day who stand in urgent need of skilled rehabilitation is so great that many receive no more than token treatment at best or none at all at worst. A tremendous amount of research has been done, particularly in the last twenty years, into the causes, precipitating factors, prevention, treatment and rehabilitation; many books have been written on the subject and detailed and carefully considered techniques of treatment based on these studies have been presented; but still we are left with the army of stroke patients I refer to as 'victims' who are condemned to a state of half-living— dependent on the state care of a geriatric unit, or dependent on members of their family, with the inevitable frustration and heartbreak that follows. I make no excuse for offering another book on this vexed subject. Most of the books obtainable have been written for the specialist in each field of rehabilitation and a text that makes sense to a specialist can be gibberish to the uninitiated. I have set out to present a simple approach to this enormous problem in the hope that it may be readily understood by all.

I have spent the last ten years making a study of the difficulties involved in this field, working with hemiplegic patients and assessing the results when using the methods offered by the experts. I have made a careful study of Proprioceptive Neuromuscular Facilitation(P.N.F.) and the patterns and techniques of treatment as offered by Margaret Knott and Dorothy Voss and I consider an understanding of their basic techniques to be a necessary part of every physiotherapist's training. I also believe that every physiotherapist who deals with hemiplegic patients ought to have read and understood the reasoned and scientific approach made to the subject by Berta Bobath in her book *Adult Hemiplegia:Evaluation and Treatment.* Also, for reference and to help towards a greater understanding of assessment with diagnostic tests, I would suggest using Professor G.F. Adams book on *Cerebrovascular Disability*—but for every physiotherapist in this field of rehabilitation there is an army of patients waiting and one expert cannot go it alone. If she tries she may very well achieve outstanding results on a small percentage of the patients that come her way while the majority are virtually passed over.

I believe there is a way. I believe the answer lies in a far greater understanding of the four main problems involved in this very specialised rehabilitation. Every member of the hospital staff must understand these problems so that all work together as a team in common understanding. With understanding the actual physical handling of the patient will be carried out along identical lines by all members of the rehabilitation team, there will be continuity of treatment with a common aim and then, and only then, will the programme of rehabilitation become truly efficient.

Believing then that the answer lies in team work, first and foremost and because the early days of treatment are vital, the nursing staff are all important. The nurse who handles the new hemiplegic patient on admission to hospital and in the very early days is the key member of any rehabilitation unit. Therefore I propose to begin with the nurse—at student level—and because at this stage in her training I do not expect her to understand the mysteries of P.N.F. patterns, loss of body image or the loss of selective movement patterns, I propose to give her a very simple introduction and hope she will take this method of treatment to a certain extent on trust in the beginning and then, as her training advances, go on to a fuller understanding of the reasoning behind her work.

It is the purpose of this book to point out as simply as possible the *four main problems involved* in the physical re-education of the stroke victim and to show all who deal with the patient the difficulties involved and how they may best deal with them.

Chapter one, on the handling of the patient in the early stages, is of vital importance, and if rehabilitation is a team activity—as I believe it must be—this is the chapter the whole team must understand. The rest of the book leads on to the other members of the team and is more technical, in places a little less easy to understand, but I will continue to present it in a fairly simple style in the hope that all members of the team may understand. The specialist in each field will find that I have over-simplified but I have done this deliberately so that all may understand something of the methods used by each unit and so that each may see the treatment as a whole with the most important member of the team—the patient—guided hopefully towards a reasonable chance and a reasonable hope of independence.

Conclusion

Rehabilitation of the adult hemiplegic is, and must be, a team activity. Then, and only then, will worthwhile results be obtained. Any unit within the team that acts separately almost invariably acts at cross-purposes to the others and the efficiency of the team as a whole is impaired. The reason for this is that various methods have been tried and are used; there is more than one school of thought on the subject, but whatever the method adopted it must be adopted by the team as a whole. One team must adopt one method. I must also emphasise that in all teams dealing with this specialised rehabilitation *the nursing staff are all important.* I hope the specialist in each field will excuse my simplification of his or her subject in my effort to carry the whole team with me.

No one person can go it alone.

2. The Nurse

Early nursing of the hemiplegic patient

To avoid confusion, throughout the text of this book let us assume that the patient is male and that all members of the rehabilitation team are female. To begin with, let us also assume that he is a left-sided stroke, bearing in mind that it is generally the right-sided stroke which has speech difficulties. This will be dealt with in a later section. Apart from any difficulty in communication, rehabilitation for either side is identical.

Very quickly the team wants to know the *cause of the stroke* and turns to the physician for an answer. Diagnosis is not easy but the good physician is usually the first to admit this. A stroke may be due to cerebral thrombosis, haemorrhage or embolism, with signs and symptoms all exactly the same except for the onset which gives some indication of the cause. In thrombosis the onset may be a matter of hours or even days while in embolism it is very sudden and in haemorrhage it can be sudden, fairly sudden, or over a few hours.

In severe cases the patient usually dies without regaining consciousness.

In about eight per cent of cases there is a brain tumour, often secondary from lung cancer.

A useful and simple classification of strokes which will help the team to understand the physician's difficulty in making an immediate diagnosis may be made in the following way:

1. *Complete;* When the patient is seen for the first time the stroke is complete.

2. *Continuing;* When the patient is seen for the first time the stroke is continuing.

3. *Stuttering;* When the patient is seen and the stroke is neither complete nor continuing it is said to be a stuttering or pseudo-stroke caused by Transient Ischaemic Attacks. (T.I.A's)

Each of these three divisions may be subdivided into two: (a) affecting the territory of the brain supplied by the vertebral-basilar artery, and (b) affecting the territory of the brain supplied by the internal carotid artery. And any of these six divisions may be due to cerebral thrombosis, haemorrhage or embolism. The clinical picture depends on which part of the brain is affected, but, even then, only a rough estimate is possible with the brain simply divided into the front or the back, and the clinical picture of the second territory can sometimes mimic the first fairly closely. It is not surprising that diagnosis is not easy. This classification is helpful because the outlook for the *complete* stroke is good while it is poor for the *continuing* and *stuttering* strokes. Also it is generally the *complete* stroke which survives and with which the rehabilitation team is concerned.

Then, again, the good physician is readily able to produce facts and figures and one of these facts in particular ought to make uncomfortable hearing for all those involved in rehabilitation. For example, he will say that for every thousand stroke victims, one half will die, one third will do well but of those third a large proportion will return to face normal living with the residual problem of a useless arm, and the remainder will stay in the community to be cared for among the severely disabled. With the *complete* stroke the outlook is good, but it is obviously not good enough. The aim of the rehabilitation team must be to alter the figures so that the numbers joining the ranks of the severely and the partially disabled will be reduced considerably. And this is certainly possible if the team are well informed and therefore efficient and ready to offer the skilled know-how that is required.

In the first place every member of the team must understand that the hemiplegic patient encounters four major problems when he attempts to perform a normal movement with an affected limb.

Put very simply he is faced with the following problems:
1. A complete loss of balance on the affected side.
2. A sensory disturbance which inhibits movement.
3. A developing extensor spasticity.
4. A complete loss of free selection of precision movements.

If the rehabilitation team fails to recognise and deal with these four major problems, lack of balance and sensory loss will persist while spasticity develops unchecked. The patient's functional loss will deteriorate still further, leading to the final picture of the severely disabled hemiplegic with his affected arm hanging in a useless position at the side of his body, fixed in flexion to give the typical synergic pattern of tonic contraction, while he walks, if, indeed, he walks at all, with the awkward swinging gait of a leg in strong extensor spasm.

In the beginning how can the nurse help? She can do a very great deal to minimise his future difficulties. She must have the skilled know-how that is necessary if she is to handle him correctly so that he is given every chance of a return to full and independent living. To have the necessary skill she must understand the four problems and she must realise that these problems come within her province and are not purely the concern of the physiotherapist. She is part of the team and she is involved. It is necessary for her to look more closely at her patients problems and to understand the solution.

1. A complete loss of balance on the affected side

This happens because he has lost his normal postual reflex mechanism on his affected side. This mechanism is taken for granted in the normally healthy person. Put simply this means he has lost his righting reactions, or the patterns of movement which we all use to turn over, to get onto hands and knees and to sit and stand up; he has lost the automatic movements which retain balance; and he has lost the fine control which changes muscle tone in relation to gravity. A baby is not born with this postual reflex mechanism, he develops it when he rolls on the floor and progresses to crawling, sitting and standing. So with our hemiplegic patient this reflex mechanism has to be re-educated by working through the infant stages and progressing from rolling to crawling to standing. If this reflex mechanism is not re-educated, he will compensate with the unaffected side and will learn to walk after a fashion but he will never again initiate movement from the affected side, his arm will remain as a useless appendage, and he will join the ranks of the severely disabled.

2. *A sensory disturbance which inhibits movement*

This happens because all movements are a direct response to sensory stimuli and are controlled and guided by sight and messages from the proprioceptors, or sensory nerve endings, of muscles, tendons and joints. There is usually some degree of sensory disturbance; it may be severe or slight but it must be taken into account. Sensory disturbance can be the most crippling disablement. As treatment progresses it may be found that sensory involvement faces our patient with his greatest hurdle. There are measures which may be taken to get over the hurdle and which we will suggest later.

3. *A developing extensor spasticity* (accompanied by forearm flexion).

This happens because of the upset in muscle tone as described above, the stronger muscle groups (or agonists) working against their weaker diagonally opposite antagonists (or opponents).This is known as the synergic pattern of tonic contraction. In the leg this pattern of spasticity is easy to understand; the muscles of extension are obviously stronger than the muscles of flexion, but in the arm it is less easy to understand and it must be understood if intelligent handling of the patient is to follow. Extensor spasticity in the shoulder is accompanied by flexion in the elbow, wrist and fingers simply because the anti-gravity (or carrying) muscles of the forearm are the stronger group. In the shoulder, extensor spasticity is understood if the size and strength of latissimus dorsi is taken into account. This muscle has its origins in the posterior part of the iliac crest and the spinous process of the lumbar and lower thoracic vertebrae. It passes obliquely upwards across the back to its insertion by a strong tendon into the floor of the bicipital groove of the humerus. Its action is to internally rotate and adduct the humerus and it also assists in *extension* of the arm at the shoulder joint (Fig. 1).

Remember that man evolved from animals. Extension must be understood. It is also helpful to remember that latissimus dorsi is sometimes referred to as the 'policeman's tip muscle'. A policeman ought not to accept a tip, and so as not to be seen to do so he holds his hand behind his back, his shoulder in extension with his arm in medial (or internal) rotation. Latissimus dorsi belongs to a strong group of depressor muscles of the shoulder which act against the weaker elevators to produce strong spasm which draws the shoulder downwards and backwards into internal rotation. Therefore, in the untreated hemiplegic we find the typical synergic pattern of tonic contraction showing this tight extension,

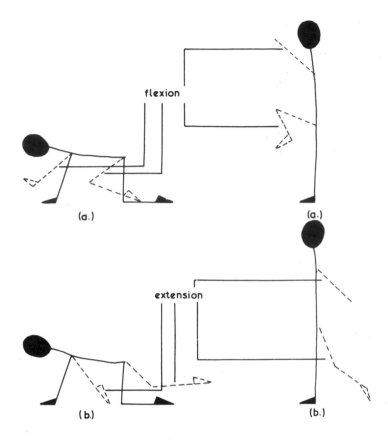

FIG.1: Explanation of flexion and extension.

adduction with internal rotation (policeman's tip position) at the shoulder with flexion (usually accompanied by pronation) of the forearm and strong extensor spasticity in the leg. Spasticity begins distally in the flexors of the fingers and plantar flexors of the toes and spreads upwards, while contraction of muscle begins proximally in the shoulder and hip. Remembering the size and origins of latissimus dorsi, we can also expect lateral shortening of the trunk muscles on the affected side.

4. *A complete loss of free selection of precision movements*

This is inevitable with the problems described in 1, 2 and 3. Where there is loss of balance, sensory loss and spasm, the ability to initiate and perform normal movements is severely or completely impaired. There may be limited movement patterns which, when used, need a great deal of effort and the effort will increase the spasm. At this point no more need be said. It will be readily seen that prevention of spasm is of first importance and balance training and sensory stimulation must be undertaken. Therefore, the members of the rehabilitation team will probably find it helpful to understand the jargon used by the expert in movement re-education. Loss of balance is referred to as loss of the *postural reflex mechanism* and sensory impairment as loss of *sensory discrimination*. We now have the complete picture. The team must not delay if they are to retrain equilibrium and sensory discrimination. But if strong extensor spasm is allowed to develop it will prevent re-education and it will make it quite impossible for the patient to initiate all normal everyday movements against this growing postural spastic pattern.

The place of the nurse in the team

In the beginning her patient may be conscious or unconscious. It is not our purpose here to enter into a discussion on the nursing skill necessary to care for an unconscious patient. This is well taken care of in the régime of any skilled medical ward. Our purpose here is to state clearly and simply the first principles involved in the active rehabilitation of the hemiplegic patient.

As stated above, *the first aim of all treatment is to prevent spasm*. Incorrect positioning while the patient lies in bed, whether he be conscious or unconscious, will inevitably lead to a build up of spasm. His affected limbs must at all times be placed away from the direction of pull of the patterns of spasticity. Therefore he is placed so that his limbs are carefully positioned in the opposing patterns of the weaker muscle groups—the leg in flexion, the arm flexed at the shoulder in external rotation with the elbow and wrist extended. If in any doubt about the position for the arm remember the action of the powerful latissimus dorsi (the policeman's tip muscle), put your own arm behind your back in internal rotation, then reverse the movement—draw your arm out from behind your back, rotate it externally and lift it forward. Thus you have the important anti-spasm pattern to be used for your patient's affected arm and the arm should be carefully maintained in this position during the initial weeks of nursing. Sometimes it is not always possible to maintain the limbs in the complete anti-spasm pattern for the entire twenty-four hours of every day. In that case, part of the pattern must be maintained and, in particular, external rotation of the humerus must be maintained at all times. Remember that side flexion of the trunk with lateral rotation of the head towards the affected side must also be prevented. N.B. The arm is lifted forwards at the shoulder in the *anatomical* position.

The following points should be noted so that correct positioning is maintained at all times while the patient lies in bed.

1. *Lying on the back,* or supine, is the position which must be used with the greatest care because it is the position which produces maximal extensor spasticity, giving retraction or a dropping backwards of the arm in internal rotation (the undesired policeman's tip position) and full extension of hip and knee with outward rotation of the leg. When supine lying cannot be avoided the paralysed shoulder and arm should be carefully placed on a pillow so that the shoulder is lifted forward—or protracted—with the arm slightly elevated in external rotation, elbow and wrist extended—the opposite position to the policeman's tip position. Similarly, a pillow is placed under the hip to prevent retraction or a dropping backwards of the pelvis and lateral rotation of the leg.

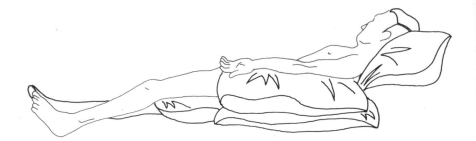

FIG. 2: Lying on the back.

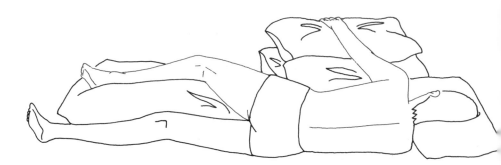

FIG. 3: Lying on the sound side

.....The knee is placed in slight flexion and, at this stage, the head is placed in lateral flexion towards the sound side (Fig. 2).

2. *Lying on the sound side* is a good position provided the patient is in full side lying and the limbs on the affected side are correctly positioned, that is, in the position which will inhibit spasm.Therefore the affected shoulder must be protracted, or brought forward, and this is simply achieved by placing the paralysed arm well forward across a supporting pillow with the elbow extended. The affected leg is placed forward in a similar position, resting on a second supporting pillow with hip and knee in a natural position of flexion (Fig. 3).

3. *Lying on the affected side* is also suitable provided care is again taken with positioning of the affected limbs. The affected shoulder must be placed well forward and the elbow extended in the supine position, that is, with the palm uppermost. The affected leg lies in a comfortable position with slight flexion of the knee. The sound leg is placed in flexion on a supporting pillow (Fig. 4).

If the nurse is in any doubt about the correct positioning she should consult the diagrams carefully. It will be noted that in every case some part, if not the whole, of the spasm inhibiting pattern is used.

If the patient is unconscious, consciousness is usually regained within a fairly short space of time; it may be minutes or hours. Generally speaking the outlook is poor if consciousness is not regained within three days. As soon as consciousness is regained our patient's active rehabilitation begins. Remember that an all important passive beginning has already been made with his correct positioning while he was unconscious and as long as he is in bed (be it only during the night) this correct positioning must continue. Correct positioning of ward furniture is also important. Our patient's bedside locker or table must be placed *on his affected side.* Also the nurse must not be misled when she examines him and finds the affected limbs are in a state of flaccid paralysis, that is the affected limbs are floppy, heavy and relaxed and give no resistance to passive movements. There is

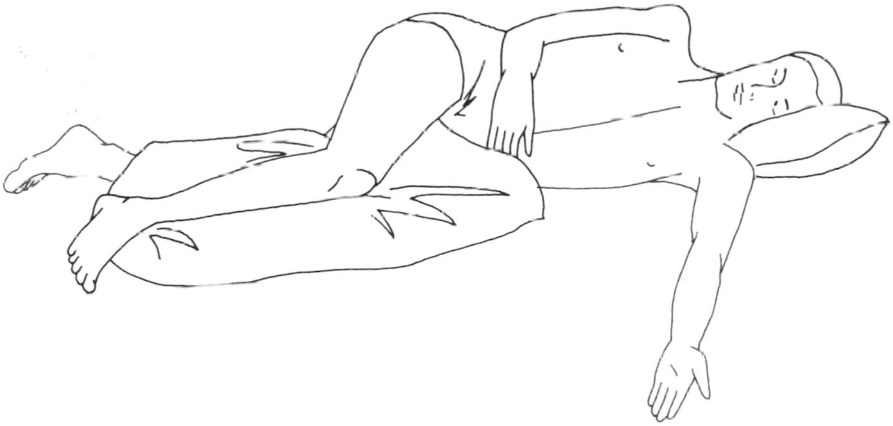

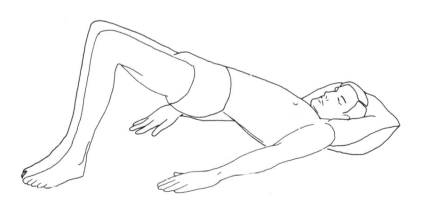

FIG.4: Lying on the affected side.

FIG.5: Bridging

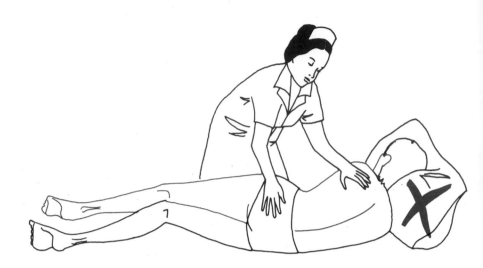

FIG.6: Rolling on to sound side (NURSE OUGHT TO HAVE REMOVED PILLOW).

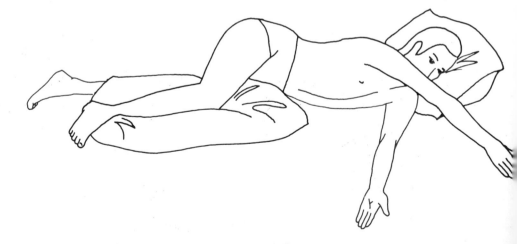

FIG.7: Rolling on to affected side.

almost always an initial stage of flaccid paralysis before the onset of spasticity and correct positioning at all stages is essential. She must remember her main aim is to prevent the development of this rigid spastic condition and it is essential to take avoiding action from the very beginning.

From a nursing point of view the best possible beginning of active mobilisation comes quite simply as part of normal ward routine and often the nurse is not aware of the positive step she is helping her patient to take towards a restoration of former voluntary activity.

Firstly, for bed-pan nursing, the patient is taught to 'bridge' (Fig. 5). Bridging consists of lying on the back with hips and knees flexed and lifting the pelvis off the bed. In the beginning the nurse will hold the affected leg in position and assist the pelvic raising. A large, awkward or confused patient may need the assistance of two nurses, one on either side of the bed with a single handgrip under the small of his back. One nurse holds the affected leg in the crook position while the other uses her free hand to place the bed-pan in position.

Secondly, for bed making purposes, the patient is taught to roll from side to side. By actively using the trunk muscles involved in this elementary exercise the patient is himself making the first voluntary movement which will lead him forward towards a return to active living. Rolling from side to side, then, is of primary importance. But, once again even for this simple exercise care must be taken not to allow the affected arm and leg to be dragged backwards to give retraction at the hip and shoulder and not to allow side flexion of the trunk. (Figs. 6 and 7). In Fig. 6 the nurse is assisting the patient to roll onto his sound side while she holds the hip and shoulder well forward in good positions but *she ought first to have removed the pillow* so as to prevent the undesirable side flexion of the trunk. When rolling onto the affected side, as in Fig. 7, the active arm and leg are thrown across the body and the affected arm and leg maintain their anti-spasm positions.

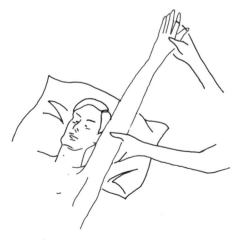

FIG. 8 (a): Arm elevation with outward rotation in supine lying.

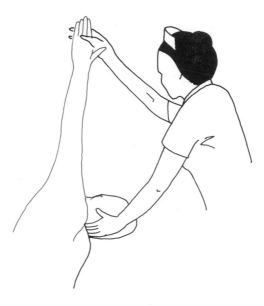

FIG 8(b): Arm elevation with outward rotation in side lying
(NOTE EXTENSION OF UPPER SPINE).

With bridging and rolling active mobilisation has begun.

The importance of bridging

This is important because the crook-lying position (lying on the back with knees flexed and held firmly together to prevent outward rotation at the hips) is the position used to inhibit build up of extensor spasm in the affected leg. The active flexion of the sound leg also helps to tilt the pelvis forwards and initiates active holding in flexion of the affected leg. Lifting the pelvis off the bed brings the trunk muscles on the affected side into action, initiating hip movement. Recovery begins proximally, that is in the hip and the shoulder, and bridging is an easy way to begin mild weight bearing on the affected leg without producing extensor spasticity. Therefore, this exercise plays an important part in preparation for standing up and sitting down. Later the mobile pelvis will be an essential part of stable rhythmical walking. Early weight bearing is a necessary and essential feature of rehabilitation if full recovery is to be obtained.

The importance of rolling

This is most important because movements of the trunk return first and, as in the case of the baby, the primitive movements involved in trunk rotation are the first to be educated. Properly controlled, the movement helps to promote awareness of both sides of the body, to relax spasticity by shoulder and hip protraction—an essential part of the spasm inhibiting patterns—and, with the rotation of the trunk, initiates active movements of the limbs. Re-education of the lost postural reflex mechanism has begun.

At this stage it should have become clearly understood why the co-operation of the nursing staff in the team's programme of rehabilitation is essential. It is of the utmost importance for the nurse to realise that the initial stage of flaccid paralysis present in the early days after a stroke need not necessarily pass on to the second stage of major spasticity. If she recognises the difficulties that will face her patient with the development of strong spasticity, and if she understands that she can play a big part in helping to re-educate a whole person, in particular by doing all she can to reduce his chance of developing strong spasticity, she will be more than ready to co-operate and become one of the key members of the team. By keeping a careful eye on correct positioning of the affected limbs so as to inhibit spasm while the patient lies in bed, by teaching rolling from side to side for bed making—without allowing retraction of the affected hip and shoulder—and by teaching the simple exercise of bridging for the easy delivery of a bed-pan *the efficient nurse has made an excellent beginning towards her patient's optimum recovery.*

It should, therefore, also be readily understood by all members of the team why bridging and rolling are frequently used in rehabilitation exercises done on a large floor mat in the physiotherapy department. But it will be impossible to proceed with these exercises in the physiotherapy department if the patient has been badly handled in the ward and has developed a retracted and painful shoulder. Nor will he be able to proceed with the subsequent series of exercises used to promote recovery. Contraction of the shoulder joint frequently holds up rehabilitation for some considerable time, if not permanently, and it can be prevented by diligent care in the early stages.

In the well organised team a physiotherapist will be on hand to supervise and guide the student nurses in the early handling of stroke patients and to demonstrate the full range of passive movements to be given several times a day. From the point of view of rehabilitation, nursing care and physiotherapy have now reached the stage where they should dovetail, and through the next steps in rehabilitation each should welcome the assistance of the other. The nurse will help by passively flexing and extending toes and ankle, fingers and wrist, knee, hip and elbow, but once again, the position of the shoulder during all movements must be carefully watched and both the leg and the arm should be kept within the pattern that inhibits spasm. Knee and hip should be bent and stretched with the ankle held at a right angle and the leg must not be allowed to go into outward rotation; the toes and ankle are moved with the leg in semiflexion. *The shoulder joint must have special care.* It must not be allowed to rotate inwards or medially. Elevation with external rotation is the arm pattern which inhibits spasm. It may be done in supine lying (lying on the back), or lying on the sound side. When it is done on the back, as the arm is raised upwards with fingers and elbow extended, it is also rotated so that the palm turns well round to face the head of the bed and the thumb points outwards towards the therapist who is standing at the edge of the bed level with her patient's head while she performs the passive movement. This arm position often leads to confusion between internal and external

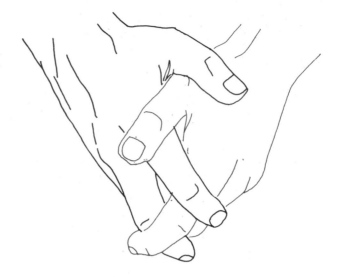

FIG.9 : Hand clasp position.

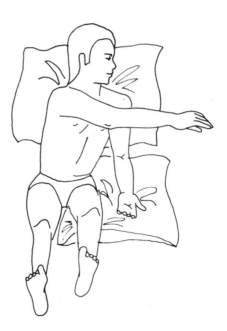

FIG.10 : Rotation of shoulders against pelvis (CROSS FACILITATION).

rotation. From the point of view of inhibition of spasm and shoulder mobilisation it is of first importance and it must be understood. When the arm reaches up over the head, palm *inwards,* the arm is in *external* rotation. To prevent any confusion, or if in any doubt about obtaining the correct position, try it on yourself. Stand with your back against a wall and touch the wall above your head with the palm of one hand and then, without allowing any rotation, lower your arm to the side of your body. It will then be quite obvious that your arm is in full external rotation, palm facing forwards and thumb pointing outwards and backwards. Note that it is not a full spiral movement. The starting position for the patient's arm is as shown in Fig. 2 with the arm already in external rotation and only a few more degrees of external rotation are obtained as the arm is elevated (Fig. 8a). When the exercise is done lying on the sound side and the arm is put through the same movement pattern, the head is tilted backwards to give extension of the upper spine which will reinforce the inhibition of spasm. This exercise makes a valuable contribution towards the prevention of painful contractures of the shoulder muscles because it is performed in the complete anti-spasm pattern (Fig. 8b).

Even although it is often not apparent at this stage, a certain degree of spasticity, however mild, will be found in all stroke patients. This is not important. The main aim is to prevent excessive spasm which leads to excessive contraction of muscles. When this begins to happen, spasm is first noticed in the flexors of the wrist and fingers and in the plantar flexors of the ankle and it spreads upwards in both limbs. As we have already said, contraction of muscle works in the reverse order, beginning proximally and spreading distally and is first particularly noticeable in the shoulder. We, as a team, must do all that we can to prevent this from happening. Our patient ought now to be taught a useful modification of the elevation in external rotation exercise for the arm. He clasps his hands (Fig. 9) in front of his body, *elbows extended,* and raises both hands above his head. Try this exercise for yourself and you will find that with both hands clasped in this position, the moment you extend your elbows the arms rotate externally at the shoulders and the shoulders are brought well forward— again the anti-spasm pattern—so that spasm is inhibited while, with double arm raising, shoulder mobility is maintained. This is often the patient's first independent exercise towards self-care.

Towards self-care

It has already been said that the patient's bedside locker or table ought to be placed on his affected side. As we are dealing with a left-sided stroke the locker or table will be placed on his left-hand side. The reasoning behind this arrangement ought now to be fully understood by the nurse. Remember that a five months fetus can rotate its head to the side that is tickled by an outside stimulus. With our patient the outside stimulus is the desire to see and to reach towards his locker and his head automatically follows his eyes. He lifts his right arm and his head forwards and sideways towards the left hip and rolls towards the locker. This may happen many times a day and, provided his left shoulder is correctly positioned, he will be making a valuable contribution towards re-establishing the function he has lost.

Before he gets up, it may be necessary for him to sit up in bed. Careful positioning is again of the utmost importance. A footboard should not be used as he will press down against it and build up extensor spasm. Instead a pillow ought to lift the affected hip slightly forward, keeping the leg from rolling into external rotation and the knee will lie comfortably in a slight degree of flexion. Now when he reaches towards his locker he rotates his shoulders against his pelvis—an important reflex-inhibiting movement against extensor spasticity—and by reaching out towards the locker with his right hand he is working through the affected side across the midline of the body and initiating bilateral activity. (Fig. 10). This type of rehabilitation is referred to as *cross facilitation*. We have already used it in rolling and it plays a major part in our programme of treatment.

Getting up

The patient should get up out of bed as soon as possible and the physician usually gives the go-ahead immediately after the initial acute period. There are four simple exercises the nurse can teach her patient at this stage. If possible, any nurse who is a newcomer to the team ought to have some instruction in these exercises from the physiotherapist. Correctly taught, the patient will learn quickly and as soon as he masters the exercises he will be able quite safely to get out of bed with little or no help. As well as assisting greatly with his rehabilitation the nurse will find she also helps herself by cutting out heavy lifting. Given a little time and patience in the beginning, the nurse quickly finds herself in a situation where she can manage her patient single-handed with the minimum of effort. Correctly handled, getting out of bed to sit in a chair is a simple, straightforward action involving one nurse and her patient. Badly handled, it takes two nurses to manhandle the patient and all three finish up looking as if they have just taken part in a rugby scrum. This takes away all dignity, initiative, self-respect and optimism from the patient and reduces his chance of successful rehabilitation considerably. There is a 'right' way to approach this stage of re-education and once it has been understood and used by the nurse she will never resort to the difficult 'wrong' way.

The right way

First position the chair and put slippers and dressing-gown within easy reach. The chair is placed alongside the bed on the patient's affected side with its back parallel with the head of the bed. I am convinced that wheelchairs, wherever possible, are to be avoided. They encourage the idea of helplessness and discourage a hopeful and positive approach to recovery and full function.

Now the patient is ready for instruction in the following four simple exercises:
1. Side lying with one-arm support
2. Sitting up
3. Training sitting balance
4. Transferring to chair.

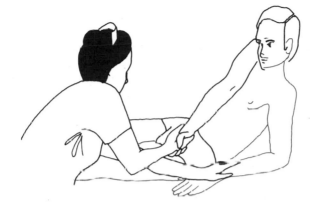

FIG.11 : Side lying with one-arm support.

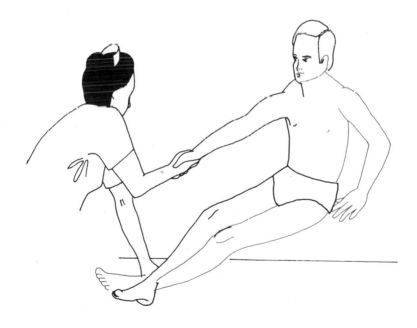

FIG. 12 : Sitting up.

Some patients will master the exercises at once; others will take longer and constant repetition is necessary; if possible each step ought to be mastered before moving on. Begin with number 1 and begin to teach it as soon as your patient reaches the stage of stretching out his right hand towards his locker.

1. *Side lying with one-arm support* (Fig. 11)

The nurse holds the patient's left elbow firmly in its resting position on the bed with her left hand and takes a firm grip of his right hand with her right hand— handshake position or cross grasp. Remember that the resting position of the arm has the shoulder well forward and the humerus externally rotated. She then assists him, with a cross pull, to raise himself onto his left elbow. If the starting position was correct the elbow will be directly below the shoulder, *not behind the shoulder,* and great care must be taken to see that shoulder retraction is not allowed. The patient should then be encouraged to balance on the elbow before he is lowered gently back onto the bed. This is repeated several times until he gets the feel of the movement. Some patients need more assistance than others; some will already have started the exercise unaided when rolling to reach the locker or table. The object of the exercise is twofold. It is the first movement towards getting up and it is an important step forward in rehabilitation. By bearing weight from elbow to shoulder on the affected side, it is a vital and integral part of the rehabilitation regime, weight being distributed from the elbow up through the shoulder joint. Remember that we have already said early weight bearing is an essential feature of treatment if full recovery is to be obtained. Also remember that by working across the midline of the body you are helping to re-educate awareness of the affected side and its position in space. You are once more making a positive move to ensure that the loss of the *postural reflex mechanism* and *sensory discrimination* do not later become major obstacles which will put an end to any reasonable hope of regaining lost function.

2. *Sitting up* (Fig. 12)

This is an easy progression from position 1. With a patient who masters the positions readily the nurse need not change her handshake grasp. She simply continues the cross pull and the patient throws his right leg across his left leg to assist the sideways turn (as he did in rolling) while the nurse supports the left leg with her left hand and lowers it down over the edge of the bed as he comes up into the sitting position. With a heavy, more difficult and confused patient it may be necessary in the beginning stages to have a second nurse standing on the far side of the bed and assisting by giving shoulder support.

Provided due care is taken to inhibit build up of muscle spasm, the success of our rehabilitation programme depends on *constant repetition of exercises* leading forward by easy progressions through a carefully planned pattern. This method of sitting up is a progression from simple rolling.

3. *Training sitting balance*

The nurse continues to stand beside the bed and in front of her patient to give him a feeling of security while she supports his shoulders with both her hands and his knees with her knees. From now on, any physical contact the nurse or any member of the team makes with her hands on the patient will be made with a little pressure, or *resistance,* which is given to re-establish balance and righting reactions. It will be referred to as *resistance* or, in the diagrams, marked by a capital R with an arrow to show the direction of pressure (Fig. 13).

In the ideal situation the correct height of bed is the height which allows the patient to sit with his knees at right angles and his feet firmly on the floor. If this is not possible a wooden box may be used as a footstool to give the same effect.

The patient is now ready for a short training session in sitting balance. The nurse gently releases the supporting pressure given by her hands. If he shows a tendency to fall sideways to the left she reinforces her supporting pressure, then increases it still further on his strong side while she decreases it on his affected side. Very soon she is able to remove one hand while she continues to give *resistance* with the appropriate hand placed firmly on her patient's strong side. It is never a pure sideways movement. The patient will show a tendency to fall sideways and backwards with rotation, or sideways and forwards with rotation, therefore the nurse supports and then *resists* and *guides* in the correct diagonal, leading him in the opposite diagonal into the upright sitting position. *This is not a difficult thing to learn.* If the patient has to develop a feeling for the exercise, so also has the nurse and she very quickly learns to feel the diagonal pattern of sideways falling and to support and then *resist* and *guide* in the correct diagonal. She is using the patient's strong side to rehabilitate the weak side. Having safely led her patient into this sitting position, he must learn to hold with his strong side against the *resistance* she offers with her hand and to remain in an upright position. The exercise should not become a battle of strength. Gently and firmly the nurse teaches the patient to *hold* against *resistance,* and finally to remain firmly upright when she slowly removes her hand. So sitting balance is established. The nurse's commands should be short and easy to understand throughout. For example: 'Push against me. Hold it! Don't let me push you over. Hold it! And now stay there.' Sometimes touch is enough and no commands are necessary. At no time should the patient be allowed to feel insecure and in danger of falling onto the floor.

Sometimes it is necessary to repeat these initial three exercises over and over again before the desired result is achieved. Training sessions should be fairly frequent and not prolonged and, in my experience, the quickest and most satisfactory results are usually obtained where treatment is started in the very early days. If the staff situation permits, a physiotherapist ought to be available to make a large contribution towards the early training in these primary and important exercises. The patient is at the most critical stage in his programme of rehabilitation. Time spent now on correct handling and training will cut down the length of time he must spend in hospital and give him a reasonable hope of

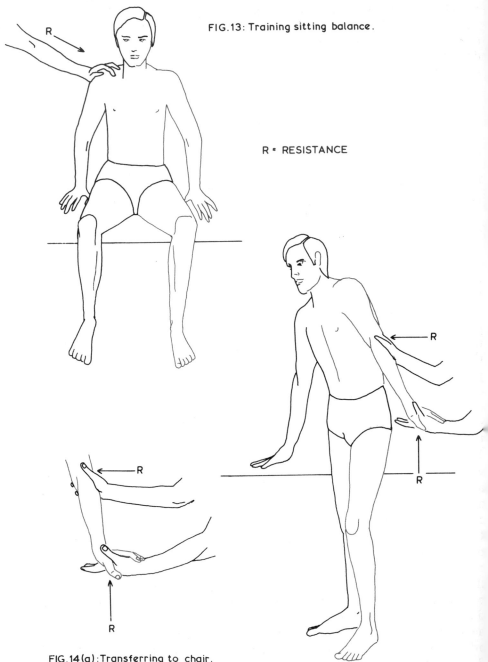

FIG.13: Training sitting balance.

R = RESISTANCE

FIG.14(a): Transferring to chair.

full functional recovery. But every nurse who deals with stroke patients ought to understand the reasoning behind these initial steps in rehabilitation and ought to be able to handle the patient accordingly.

As soon as he has learnt to sit on the edge of the bed with his sitting balance established—or well on the way to becoming established—it is time to put on his dressing-gown. This saves wrestling with it while he is lying in bed or when he is sitting in his chair. He may need help in the beginning; the nurse must not let frustration build up nor yet cramp his style. He must be allowed to do as much as possible for himself. The left or paralysed arm goes into the gown first. The slippers should not be put on at this stage. Bare feet on a cold floor give a feeling of security because there is no danger of slipping and recovery of active sensory discrimination is also given a boost; this should be taken on trust if it is not yet understood. It is as well to remember that the patient may be diabetic and, if so, bare feet and a dirty floor are undesirable because any infection in a small skin crack could lead to major gangrene.

4. *Transferring to chair* (Fig. 14a)

Again it is often surprising how easily this progression is made if steps 1 to 3 have been carefully taught. The chair must be in the correct position so that all that is required of the patient is one easy movement. Standing up and sitting down with a quarter turn to the right. He places his right hand firmly on the bed, leans on it with an extended elbow, raises his buttocks and pivots a quarter turn to lower his buttocks onto the waiting chair. If necessary support may be given by the nurse through the left hand and arm as illustrated in Fig. 14a. This is a good position, weight being distributed from the palm of the hand through the extended elbow and up to the shoulder which is held in external rotation. It is one of the arm rehabilitation exercises which the physiotherapist will use frequently in her treatment programme. If, however, the patient proves a little more difficult to handle, the second method of transferring to a chair ought to be used (Fig. 14b). Here the nurse gives her patient considerably more support, using her knees against his and supporting his trunk with her left arm while she supports his affected arm with her right hand cupped under his elbow. The arm must not be allowed to hang in internal rotation. To add to his feeling of security he is encouraged to lean forward and place his sound arm firmly round his nurse. Leaning forward is a necessary part of standing up and leaning forward is a posture which generally has to be re-educated, but I have not come across any patient who is unable to transfer to a chair using this second method. As soon as the transfer is safely accomplished a further short training session in sitting balance will help to prevent lounging or falling sideways in the chair. Now it is time to put his slippers on. While he is sitting up, care should be taken by the nurse to see that he maintains a good position. When necessary, a little pressure or *resistance* gently applied diagonally on the right place will gain a *response* and the patient will straighten up. If in any doubt about the correct positions for the bed, chair and locker, consult Fig. 15.

To put the patient back to bed the whole process is repeated in reverse.

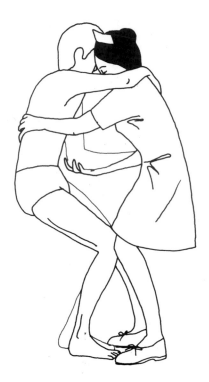

FIG. 14(b): Transferring to chair (less stable patient).

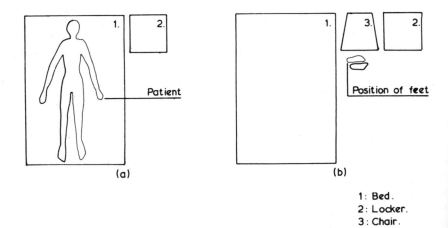

Patient

Position of feet

(a)   (b)

1: Bed.
2: Locker.
3: Chair.

FIG.15: Position of furniture {(a)Patient in bed.
                              {(b)Patient getting up.

Getting out of bed to use the commode should now be a relatively simple exercise provided the commode is correctly positioned alongside the bed. Or, transferring from chair to commode is simply a matter of training the patient to lean forward, place his right hand firmly on the bed, and stand while the chair is pulled out of position and the commode slipped in. In all such operations support should be given to the affected arm, the nurse placing her hand firmly in position below the elbow and supporting the forearm, or, when possible, using the grip as illustrated in Fig. 14a. The arm must never be allowed to hang from the shoulder in internal rotation. (Consult Figs. 16 and 17)

A suitable chair for the hemiplegic patient is illustrated in Fig. 18a. There are a great many unsuitable chairs on the market and care should be taken to make the right choice. It should have a broad base, solid forearm supports, a comfortably upright back and be virtually impossible to tip. It should be used in conjunction with the right table, that is, a table with a brake to lock the wheels and adjustable height as illustrated in Fig. 18b. The table can then be placed and locked in position in front of the patient at the correct height to support his forearms. He should be encouraged to lean forward with his weight equally distributed on both arms and he should be taught to practice exercising in this position, transferring his weight from arm to arm while making sure that the forearm on the affected side does not turn inwards but points straight forwards with wrist and fingers extended and thumb abducted. Thus he maintains the anti-spasm position with the humerus externally rotated while weight is transferred from elbow to shoulder. This is a valuable rehabilitation exercise and, if he can be taught to do it on his own, it makes another step forward in self-care.

The nurse has now made a major and essential contribution towards her patient's rehabilitation. She has tackled the whole problem with an approach that will rebuild his confidence in himself and she has helped him to take the first steps towards a reasonable hope of regaining his initiative and independence. There is, however, another aspect for her to consider. She may have to handle a right-sided stroke and therefore a patient with communication difficulties which may involve difficulty in articulation or in understanding, or both. In that case it is to be hoped the nurse first gets used to handling the patient who has no speech difficulty. Later she will have gained a feeling for her work and she will begin to find she can handle both types of case equally well, using *resistance* (or hand pressure) to elicit the *response* she needs for each progression she has to make.

There is no time to lose if emotional distress is to be minimised. The enormity of the shock the patient has suffered is hard to imagine. Suddenly his body refuses to obey him and he may not be able to make himself understood. At worst, he may not even be able to understand what is said—although, fortunately, the latter condition is not so common, and it is as well for the nurse to remember that in most cases her patient's understanding is unimpaired. Constant reassurance is necessary, frustration must be avoided and never at any time should members of the rehabilitation team talk across his bed as if he was not there. The aim from the beginning is centered on his return to normal living and he himself must do most of the work towards this end, but this will only be

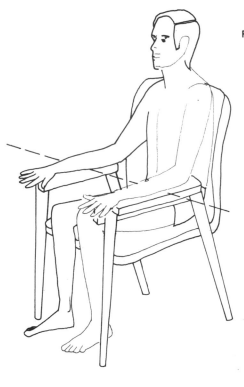

FIG. 16 : The right way.

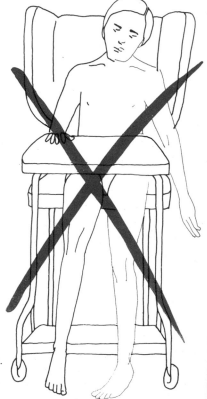

FIG. 17: The WRONG way.

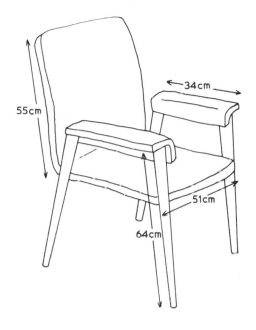

FIG.18(a): Suitable chair.

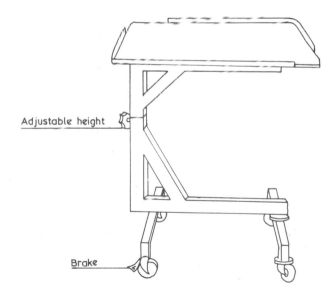

FIG.18(b): Suitable table.

possible if he is shown what has to be done by competent and understanding helpers.

However slow he is and however time-consuming it seems for the staff who stand by, he must be encouraged to do things for himself provided he works within the limits of frustration. With a return of self-confidence and independence the end result will more than justify the time taken to achieve it. We are all vulnerable. The youngest adult stroke patient I have treated in recent years was twenty-three.

When the patient's speech is disturbed he must be treated with the greatest care. There are three main types of language disorder and, in the beginning, it is not always possible to distinguish one from the other. If we are lucky we will have a speech therapist in our team. Speech therapy is a highly specialised skill which requires an expertise that is only acquired with specific training, and it is probably least understood by the other experts in the team. Unfortunately, speech therapy is not yet available in every team. I have included a short section on speech difficulty and I hope the specialist will forgive my simplification in an attempt to give a few points which will make for better understanding all round. If separate departments within the team do not understand the jargon used in other departments, what hope is there of complete understanding of the patient's problems and of a reasonable continuity of treatment. I suggest the nurse refers to this section and, in the beginning, while she is gaining an understanding and insight into the difficulties involved for her patient, I cannot stress too strongly that she must always remember not to talk across him as if he was not there; there is no reason to assume that he cannot hear or understand all that is said. Shouting at him will not make her meaning clearer, it will only confuse, depress and anger him. The brain's power of thought is usually untouched and after coming to terms with the dreadful shock and humiliation of suddenly finding himself a helpless invalid—which, in the beginning, he is—his mental activity is unimpaired. *A breakdown in communication does not usually mean a breakdown in comprehension.*

A positive approach to early nursing of the stroke patient has been given. So far, the nurse has had more to do with the patient's welfare than any other member of the team. The physiotherapist is also involved from the very early days, her programme of treatment dovetailing with the nursing team, their methods of handling similar from the beginning. Constant repetition is required; not constant confusion because no two members of the team handle the patient in the same way. One team must use one method and no one person can go it alone. There can be no rigid barriers between departments; the physiotherapist moves freely round the wards and as soon as the physician indicates that the patient is ready to be taken to the physiotherapy department, the nurse ought to be encouraged to 'sit in' at some of the treatment sessions there and she ought to learn more about the reasoning behind the method of treatment used. Continuity of treatment is of primary importance, and for continuity of understanding we must follow our male, left-sided, *complete* stroke from the ward to the physiotherapy department and find out what happens there.

3. The Physiotherapist

Physiotherapy for the hemiplegic patient

Physiotherapy of a very high standard must be offered to the hemiplegic victim if he is not to spend the rest of his days with a useless arm hanging at his side and to move about with the awkward swinging gait of tight trunk muscles and a leg in extensor spasm. It should now be fairly obvious to all members of the hemiplegic rehabilitation team that there are two main aims in treatment which must be borne in mind twenty-four hours a day—twenty-four hours, bearing in mind that as far as possible he ought to be correctly positioned and supported by pillows at night so that he sleeps with his affected limbs placed away from the direction of pull of the patterns of spasticity (Figs. 2, 3 and 4.). The two main aims in treatment are intimately bound up with each other, are equally important, and to promote satisfactory recovery they must never be forgotten. The first is to prevent the development of excessive contraction of spastic muscles and the second is to re-educate former full function. Without the first the second is impossible.

All through the initial steps in rehabilitation the physiotherapy staff and the nursing staff must work in close co-operation and it is up to the senior physiotherapist and the clinical instructor to keep a watchful eye on the maintenance of correct positioning and to give advice where necessary. The senior physiotherapist ought to be prepared to help junior and less experienced members of the team towards a fuller understanding of the problems involved and the reasoning behind the techniques used. With complete co-operation, not only is teaching of younger members of all departments not resented, it is expected and received with enthusiasm.

The jargon used by the physiotherapist sometimes confuses the other members of the rehabilitation team and leads to a breakdown in communication and therefore, because of misunderstanding, to lack of continuity of treatment between departments. We have discussed the four main problems the patient encounters. Put very simply these are:

1. Balance loss
2. Sensory loss
3. Movement loss
4. Developing spasticity

All are negative factors except the developing spasticity and the first aim of all treatment is to prevent this. *In the hemiplegic patient where there is balance loss and sensory loss movement cannot be performed.* This suggests a simple equation:

Balance loss + Sensory loss = **Movement loss** + **Developing spasticity**, remembering that with loss of movement on the affected side, the strong muscle groups go into spasm against their weaker antagonists. With all hemiplegics there is some degree of spasm, however mild, and if it is allowed to develop, as it inevitably will unless the correct precautions are taken, within a year to eighteen months after onset contraction of spastic muscles will eventually inhibit all potential activity of the weaker antagonists.

Again, getting right down to the basic facts, the serious problems involved in re-educating the hemiplegic patient can be clearly seen and understood if simple terms are used.

Balance loss + sensory loss must be re-educated, and then, and only then, movement loss may be re-established and developing spasm will cancel out, providing developing spasm has been held at a minimum all through the programme of rehabilitation. Therefore, from the day of onset of hemiplegia we are dealing with one problem, the problem of spasm. In other words, the four main problems in the rehabilitation of the hemiplegic patient can now be seen as one. We are left with the relatively simple problem of *preventing muscle spasm while balance loss and sensory loss are re-established.* It is a simple problem because there is an answer and if the problem is understood the straightforward and possible solution is also understood.

All members of the rehabilitation team will now understand the importance of the part the nurse plays towards the prevention of developing muscle spasm by careful and correct positioning and handling of her patient. While discussing the handling of the patient in the physiotherapy department, and in order that all departments should understand something of the meaning behind the language the physiotherapist uses, a step by step explanation will be given.

1. *Balance loss*

As we have already said, our hemiplegic patient has lost his *normal postural reflex mechanism* on the affected side. He was not born with this mechanism, he developed it after birth in the infant stages of kicking, rolling, crawling, kneeling and standing. When fully developed this reflex mechanism has three distinct functions. Firstly, it includes the automatic postural reaction—or righting reaction—which allows him to change position smoothly and rapidly, for example from lying supine to getting into the upright position; secondly, it includes the equilibrium reaction which gives changes in muscle tone to allow him to adjust smoothly to changes in his centre of gravity; and thirdly, it includes an automatic postural adjustment to adapt to changes in gravity pull which makes for smooth movement in any action carried out in the direction of gravity, the antagonistic muscles doing the work, that is, contracting and 'paying out' slowly to control the movement. This also happens in any quick reaction where equilibrium has to be maintained against sudden movement such as maintaining balance after stumbling. It can be seen then that, to some extent, all three of these reactions overlap with alterations in muscle tone and it is quite easy to understand that with complete loss of this normal postural reflex mechanism *the balance of muscle tone is upset* (e.g. flexor tone increases in the arm) and the stronger muscles go into a permanent state of contraction (or spasticity). Normal and voluntary movement patterns cannot be performed on the affected side.

2. *Sensory loss*

This is known as loss of *sensory discrimination*. All movements result from outside sensory stimulation by way of *sight, hearing* and *touch*. Movements are guided by sight and through the stimulation of the proprioceptors of muscles, tendons and joints which are activated by movement in the tissues. Proprioceptors are sensory nerve endings receptive of sensory stimuli. Sensory stimuli, therefore, initiate and direct motor function. With sensory loss there is difficulty in initiating movement and consequent malfunction or loss of function. With any degree of loss of proprioceptive sense there is also loss of body image, body image being the ability to feel a limb, to appreciate the movements of the joints and to appreciate its place in space and its relationship to the body. The sense of touch is frequently impaired and size, shape and texture of an object held in the hand may be difficult or impossible to determine while slight variations in temperature, between warm and hot or cool and cold, are difficult to detect, although this does not usually apply to extreme variations.

In the hemiplegic patient it has long been thought that this loss of *sensory discrimination* tends to recover more readily in the leg than in the arm and a possible explanation has been given which suggests that, however severe the stroke, this is because the leg is used to some extent in early weight bearing. This would seem to suggest at once that the arm in the hemiplegic patient ought to be made to bear weight as soon as possible after the onset of the stroke. The prevention of developing spasm and early weight bearing from the palm of the hand up through an extended elbow to an externally rotated shoulder play an equally important part in retraining normal function in the arm. We can no longer accept the theory that assumes: 'Most patients on intensive treatment will walk again. Comparatively few will recover a useful hand.' Already the nurse has used the arm for weight bearing, full-arm (Fig. 14a), and half-arm, elbow to shoulder, when the patient sits correctly positioned at a table leaning on his elbows with his forearms *pointing straight forward*. The rehabilitation team must hold this principle of early weight bearing constantly in mind. Using this principle from the beginning, arm recovery ought to move forward as rapidly as leg recovery; indeed, why not more rapidly? It will shortly be shown that bearing weight through the arm using the whole of the anti-spasm pattern is easily practised, while standing on the leg uses the pattern of extensor spasticity. This would seem to suggest that deficient muscle tone in the arm ought to be more readily restored. If the arm is not being rehabilitated, where are we going wrong?

It ought to be possible to rehabilitate the stroke victim and worthwhile results ought to be obtained. The physiotherapist has an important part to play and she ought to be the prime mover in any scheme of rehabilitation, making sure that she understands the problems her patient faces and leading him forward with a hopeful attitude, because, properly handled, the outlook is hopeful.

Conclusion

In the hemiplegic patient where there is always loss of the normal postural reflex mechanism and where there is usually some degree of loss in sensory discrimination movement cannot be performed. Loss of the postual reflex mechanism means that righting reactions, equilibrium reactions, and muscle tone are all affected and with sensory loss there is difficulty in initiating and sustaining normal movement. Together, this adds up to paralysis with spasm on the affected side, and this, as we have already said, is termed the synergic pattern of tonic contraction which gives the typical hemiplegic picture. In more sophisticated language we have reached the same conclusion as before. All our treatment is aimed at re-educating these functions while we do not allow major spasticity to develop and we are then able to re-establish the normal movement which will in turn establish normal muscle tone.

Without treatment, the patient will compensate to a certain extent with the unaffected side and this will lead to walking—if he succeeds in walking—with a leg held stiffly in extension while his arm remains a useless appendage and *he will never again initiate movement from the affected side.* He becomes at best a member of the community who is trying to face normal living with the residual problem of a spastic gait and a useless arm, or he is forced to opt out of normal life and he becomes an inmate of an institution, joining the ranks of the severely diabled.

If this introduction to physiotherapy has been largely a repetition of what has gone before, then so is treatment. The only way to rehabilitate a hemiplegic patient is by constant repetition and, as we decided in the beginning, by every member of the team understanding and therefore handling the patient in a correct and similar way. As the infant developed his postural reflex mechanism, so must our patient, by rolling, crawling, kneeling and standing, while, at the same time, sensory discrimination is facilitated. Sensory loss is the most serious factor and where it is severe extra measures must be taken. The skill of the physiotherapist lies in her ability to retrain her patient, while, at all times, she uses the anti-spasm patterns, preventing the development of contraction of spastic muscles until he is able to *initiate movement from the affected side.* Brought down to these simple basic principles,it is quite easy for all members of the rehabilitation team to understand the aims of treatment, and treatment itself becomes a relatively simple exercise which ought not to present any obscure or difficult problems and which ought to be comparatively straightforward.

Suggested outline of physiotherapy treatment for hemiplegia

Having brought our male, left-sided complete stroke to the physiotherapy department our first task is to assess his condition before continuing with the programme of treatment. He has been well cared for in the ward from the day of admission and he is capable, with help, of rolling from side to side, of bridging, of propping himself on his left elbow with correct positioning, but he has not achieved independence in any of these exercises. He has achieved a fair degree of sitting balance but standing balance is poor. The arm seems to be completely flaccid but demonstrates flexor spasm in the fingers when strong stretch is applied and held, and there is mild resistance to full passive movement of the shoulder. The arm feels abnormally heavy when it is lifted by the physiotherapist and shows lack of postural tone, or complete lack of any postural reaction. Passive flexion of hip and knee meet with mild resistance when he lies supine and extension with inversion of the ankle in the typical spastic pattern is found to be present, again when strong stretch is applied and held. The prognosis ought to be good but we find a fair degree of sensory involvement. As we might expect from the picture of a severely flaccid arm and a considerably less flaccid leg, a degree of loss of sensory discrimination is present in the lower limb while it is severe in the upper limb. As far as successful rehabilitation is concerned, sensory loss presents a tremendous hurdle, but it must be regarded as a hurdle and not as a barrier and a way *must* be found to get over it.

Where proprioceptive sense, or the sense of muscular position, is impaired *we must step up the level of sensory input.* Loss of proprioception is tested by passive movements of the index finger and big toe. The patient watches the movement. Then his eyes are covered and he is asked to say if each movement is 'up' or 'down'. If he is uncertain, or he does not know, the larger joints are tested. Or, still without using his eyes, he is asked to grasp the thumb of the affected hand while the physiotherapist changes the thumb's position. Cutaneous sensibility must also be assessed and two point discrimination is used, the test depending on the patient's ability to distinguish two points from one on the finger pulps without using eyesight. Or tests in *stereognosis* may fail. These are tests where objects held in the hand are recognised by touch without using eyesight. Where there is failure in any or all of these tests the level of sensory input must be stepped up.

A satisfactory answer to this problem is found by using a pressure splint.

The patient is placed in supine lying, correctly positioned with his arm placed in slight elevation and external rotation at the shoulder, and the elbow, wrist and fingers are extended to include supination with abduction of the thumb. The leg is placed in the anti-spasm position of comfortable semi-flexion with a pillow preventing external rotation. Maintaining this position, the arm is put in a half arm, orally inflated pressure splint (Fig. 19) and then the head pillow is removed to give extension of the upper spine. The patient may be left to lie quite comfortably in this position for twenty minutes. Sensory discrimination in the leg may also be given a boost by applying a foot and ankle pressure splint. As we said before, the arm is in the *anatomical* position with the splint resting on a pillow keeping the shoulder well forward. The importance of this position cannot be stressed too often. It is the complete spasm inhibiting pattern and the earlier it is used after onset of the stroke the better, even although the arm seems to be completely flaccid.

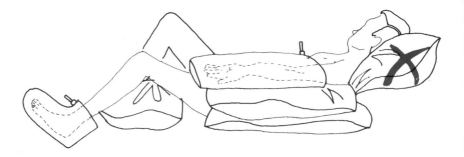

FIG. 19: Arm and leg in orally inflated pressure splints.

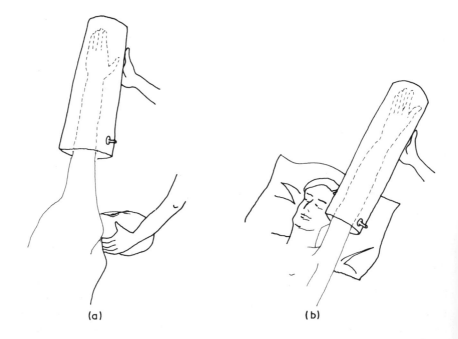

(a)   (b)

FIG. 20(a&b): Shoulder girdle maintains full range of movement.
Active assisted exercise.

Orally inflated splints are made of clear plastic casing forming a double cover. When fitted to a limb and blown up, pneumatic cushioning conforms to the shape of the limb, holding it immobile and suspended to give full support with even pressure. The splint is X-ray transparent and was originally designed as an emergency pressure splint for first-aid and safe transport of fractured, crushed or sprained limbs. As used for the hemiplegic patient it serves a double purpose.

1. *It re-educates sensory discrimination.* Pressure on the tissues bombards the proprioceptors of muscles, tendons and joints. Sustained pressure has a positive effect on loss of body image and loss of sense of touch.

2. *It inhibits muscle spasm* by holding the limb firmly in the anti-spasm pattern. The key points of spasm control in the arm, are neck, spine, shoulder girdle, wrist and fingers. With the positioning described above and the addition of the orally inflated splint to maintain wrist and finger extension, all key points are activated simultaneously. Hence the immediate comfort the splint gives with quite spectacular control of any spastic resistance. In the foot, sensory stimulation supplied by the splint along the plantar aspect helps in the re-education of active dorsiflexion of the foot and again the splint assists in the maintenance of the anti-spasm pattern (Fig. 19).

In *Case 1,* the patient as described and assessed above, pressure splints would play a large part in re-education of sensory loss. There are, however, two more cases which we must consider.

In *Case 2,* let us suppose that on arrival for the first time in the physiotherapy department we find the degree of flaccidity usually present in the new hemiplegic (and usually present in a marked degree where there is sensory loss) is no longer present and, in spite of careful nursing, the patient is developing strong spasticity. Once more the physiotherapist must move into action fast and once more the orally inflated pressure splint will prove invaluable. In this case the splint is obviously used because it *inhibits muscle spasm* as described above.

In *Case 3,* let us suppose our hemiplegic patient has reached the physiotherapy department having been admitted to hospital with residual disability some considerable time after onset and he demonstrates the typical synergic pattern of tonic contraction (extension in the leg and flexion in the arm) which prevents re-education of the postural reflex mechanism and inhibits motor function. The weakness present in the flexors of the leg and the extensors of the arm is the weakness imposed by the strong spastic agonists. With the help of the pressure splint *it is not too late to give treatment.* In Case 3, pressure splints *must* play an important part if arm spasm is to be controlled—and spasm control is the key to successful treatment. Where necessary, ice or tapping of the palm and brisk brushing with the finger-tips down the anterior aspect of the forearm should be used to relax wrist and finger spasm so that the splint may be applied with the hand in the correct position.

Only orally inflated splints are used. The warmth of the breath makes the inner plastic sheath pliable so that it moulds satisfactorily to the limb to give an all over even pressure without severe compression. The pressure splint should be used for the leg with discretion, making sure there is no underlying contra-indication, and if in doubt the physiotherapist will consult the pnysician. The knee will not be included; the leg is positioned in the anti-spasm flexion pattern and the foot and ankle are enclosed as in a boot. Treatment for the arm is of first importance. The splints should be used for two twenty minute periods daily in the physiotherapy department under supervision. Each session is immediately followed by a scheme of exercises which will be done firstly while the splints are still in position and secondly as soon as they are removed. Movements should be followed by the eyes.

Mobility of the shoulder girdle is noticeably facilitated when the spastic resistance of the scapula muscles is at its lowest with the half arm pressure splint on (Fig. 20). Arm elevation with outward (external) rotation in side lying on the sound side and in supine lying is given, making it an active assisted exercise in the beginning, and as muscle strength grows resistance is gradually given. The shape and size of the splint make it necessary for the physiotherapist to *assist* and *guide* the movement at first and later she *resists* and *guides*. Again it is not a full spiral and diagonal pattern; external rotation of the shoulder must be maintained in all positions of the arm and the degree of rotation during the performance of the exercise is minimal. In side lying extension of the upper spine is encouraged and *resistance* applied to the back of the head to reinforce the inhibition of spasm. Exponents of P.N.F. patterns and techniques must remember that in this instance the correct 'groove' for elevation of the hemiplegic arm is with minimal spiral and diagonal pattern. In other words, where the spiral and diagonal P.N.F. patterns of facilitation move into the area of the synergic patterns of tonic contraction they are not suitable for rehabilitation in hemiplegia. However, the basic techniques of P.N.F. ought to be understood by the physiotherapist and used judicially.

While the patient lies on his sound side with the half arm pressure splint still in position he is next encouraged to move the arm forwards and upwards, this time in an obvious diagonal while external rotation of the shoulder joint is maintained and increased, the physiotherapist supporting and guiding the splint. This is followed by a movement in full range, flexion to extension of the shoulder joint and once more the important external rotation is maintained.

Finally, with the splint still in position and the arm held forwards with the shoulder still in external rotation, alternate pulling and pushing movements are applied by the physiotherapist to the splint to give traction and approximation of the shoulder joint. *Traction* will promote *motor response* while *approximation* will stimulate *postural reflexes*. Both stimulate the proprioceptive centres supplying the joint structures.

All exercises are repeated with the splint off, preferably as soon as the splint is taken off, and the physiotherapist uses hand holds to keep the patient's arm in the correct anti-spasm pattern. Thumb abduction must not be forgotten and extension of the wrist and fingers with abduction of the thumb is held while approximation is applied to the shoulder through the palm of the hand and a straight elbow. The patient should be encouraged to watch what is done and to follow movements with his eyes.

Side lying on the sound side is the most suitable position for the initial leg

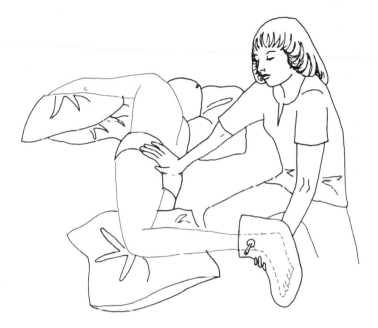

FIG.21:Side lying, hip extended,active assisted flexion and extension of the knee.

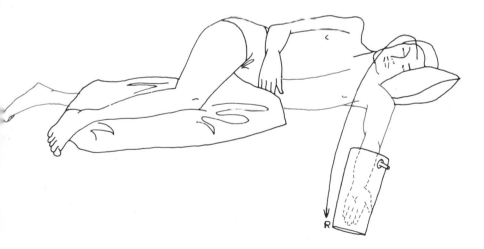

FIG.22: Side lying,active assisted flexion and extension of elbow.

exercises. The pressure splint maintains dorsiflexion of the foot and the physiotherapist assists the patient in re-education of *hip and knee flexion*. For example, she holds his knee in flexion and actively assists in flexion of the hip, leading into *resisted* flexion. Knee movement is carried out with the hip in extension (Fig. 21). Again the foot is held in dorsiflexion by the splint. *Assisted* flexion of the knee leads to *active assisted* flexion and then to *resisted* flexion. Note that while the leg exercises are given the affected arm is carefully positioned across a pillow in the anti-spasm pattern.

Again the exercises are repeated with the splint off.

Side lying on the affected side is a useful position for re-education of elbow extension (Fig. 22). The sound leg is thrown across the affected leg to give the reflex-inhibiting movement against extensor spasticity in the affected leg, and the affected leg is placed in a comfortable position of slight flexion. The affected hand is placed in a hand and wrist pressure splint and the elbow is flexed with the hand moving towards the forehead as shown in Fig. 22. *Elbow extension* is taught in this position, again moving through the stages of *assisted* and *active assisted,* until *resisted* movement is finally established.

Thus the use of the pressure splint which started as a necessary aid to the successful re-education of sensory loss is now seen to be a necessary aid to all successful treatment. In particular it gives a positive solution to the age-old problem of the residual hemi-arm. If this has not been understood, remember that the pressure exerted on the tissues stimulates the proprioceptors (sensory) and breaks down the synergic pattern of tonic contraction, maintaining the anti-spasm pattern and balancing muscle tone, making it possible to activate the antagonists (motor). Precision movements of the hand inevitably follow as treatment progresses.

Sensory loss is the most serious handicap but we must not forget that *all* hemiplegic patients have lost the *postural reflex mechanism* on the affected side and unless this is re-educated these patients will never again initiate *normal* motor patterns from the affected side. We move on to the very necessary part the physiotherapist must play in re-educating the lost postural reflex mechanism— while at the same time she continues to prevent developing spasticity—and we find, as we might by now expect, that the steps she takes to achieve her purpose also assist in recovery of any sensory loss. In other words, all through treatment, sensory loss and the postural reflex mechanism are rehabilitated simultaneously and for those members of the rehabilitation team who fail to understand fully the separate distinctions it is enough to follow the sequence of treatment which takes care of both functions while spasm-inhibiting patterns are employed at all times.

In the assessment of the patient, age and general state of health must be taken into consideration, but, whatever the age, the *postural reflex mechanism cannot be rehabilitated* without moving through the infant stages of rolling, crawling and kneeling. For the elderly it may be helpful to use a double breadth of plinth, or two plinths bolted together, for initial steps in treatment. A large floor mat, firm with a friction free surface, gives the ideal situation and also disposes of any fear of falling. If the patient has been properly handled and trained in the initial stages in the ward, getting from a chair to the floor does not present any

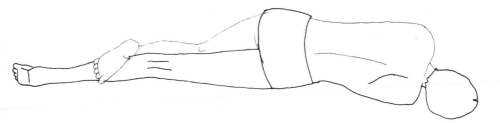

FIG. 23: Rolling, shoulder protracted, knee flexed.

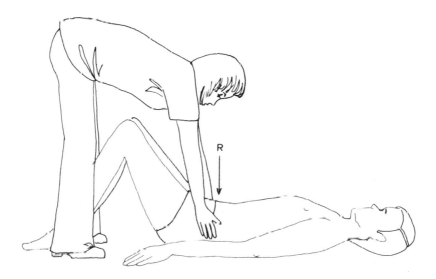

FIG. 24: Bridging against resistance.

problems. Provided the physiotherapy department is heated adequately the whole routine, including pressure splint treatment, may take place on the floor mat. Pillows for positioning where necessary ought to be available and a blanket or rug will be necessary for rest periods. Feet should be bare and a minimum of clothing worn. Skin contacts should be used where possible when handling the patient. The P.N.F. principle of stepping up *demand* by skin contact, firm handling and clear commands should be used where necessary. The patient should also be taught to follow limb movements with his eyes.

Now, let us go back to the development of movement in the baby. Motor development in the baby is from head to foot in direction, that is proximal to distal, or neck and shoulders before the arm and hand; trunk and hip before the leg and foot. He is born with motor function, the fetus develops reflex movements and in man these movements are called primitive. After birth development of motor function continues from proximal to distal and the first movements are still primitive—head turning, eye movements, kicking, finger grasp and so on. Most of us at some time have watched the infant in wonder and we have noticed these restless, primitive movements. Most of us have seen his reaction to each new development he makes. He learns to roll. Rolling is a new movement. He repeats it again and again as if he is practising his new trick—as, indeed, he is. The *primitive* or *reflex* movement he was born with becomes controlled movement which he can perform deliberately or automatically. Soon, rolling from supine to prone becomes a controlled and delicate movement to be used to lead him into crawling. In other words he has established postural and righting reactions by constant repetition of rolling, mainly because of the constant alteration of the position of his head in space and in relation to the trunk and limbs, or vice versa. Rolling leads to sitting and sitting to standing and to holding these positions. Rolling leads to crawling and crawling to walking. Therefore, rolling leads to controlled and stable walking.

Without this establishment of righting reactions (which our hemiplegic patient has lost on the affected side) there can be no controlled and delicate movement and no controlled posture. So our patient must learn to roll and he must repeat the exercise over and over again, as did the baby, our purpose being to promote optimum recovery of controlled and deliberate movement and posture. Within the limits of fatigue treatment should be intensive.

Rolling

The baby who is hampered by tight clothing and confined space builds up frustration and expends a great deal of energy to no purpose while the baby who is dressed in the minimum of clothing and given clear space develops with little effort. In our patient's case we must not allow excess effort to build up spasm. Re-education of the postural reflex mechanism demands constant repetition but effort is not necessary; it is the constant alteration of the position of his head in space and in relation to his trunk and limbs that is responsible for primitive movements once more becoming controlled. He will turn with comparative ease onto the affected side but the affected arm must be carefully positioned (Fig. 7). To roll back onto the sound side he leads with his eyes and his head (as in the development of the baby), the sequence of movement being eyes, neck, shoulders, arms, hands, trunk, legs and feet. It turns a rather difficult manoeuvre into a relatively simple one if he is taught to clasp his hands in front of his body in elevation, and the sound side assists the affected side with shoulder rotation which is followed by quick trunk rotation, legs following. The hand clasp position also prevents the affected arm from falling backwards and inwards into the forbidden spasm pattern.

In the beginning the physiotherapist may find it necessary to assist the patient's affected leg to follow the trunk rotation with the knee held in flexion, but very soon she will find that her patient can perform the movement without help.

Remembering that rotation between shoulders and pelvis is an important reflex-inhibiting pattern against extensor spasticity it is easy to understand this natural sequence of movement. Also remembering that simultaneous extension of the affected hip, knee and ankle must be avoided at all times, we rely on this reflex-inhibiting action of rolling to re-establish righting reactions without increasing extensor spasticity in the affected leg. Where treatment is started in the early days, rolling with both knees in slight flexion is easily established.

In the first visit to the physiotherapy department, rolling from side to side may be as far as the active treatment goes. This exercise should be completely and correctly mastered before continuing. It is of the utmost importance to spend time and care on this exercise. It must not be allowed to become a haphazard routine. It is *the* vital exercise in the re-education of the *postural reflex mechanism*. Every member of the team by now understands that no true rehabilitation is possible without it. All team members will also understand why it must be performed with the maintenance of correct positioning throughout. The postural reflex mechanism is being re-established *without building up spasm,* any sensory loss is being re-established *without building up spasm,* and the end result will be *balanced muscle tone* (and therefore cancellation of muscle spasm) with optimum recovery of controlled and deliberate movement. With the use of rolling the physiotherapist should also understand that any sensory loss will also be rehabilitated by movement of tissues acting on the proprioceptors or, in this instance, by bombardment of the proprioceptors by constant repetition of an exercise in cross facilitation. Once again we are rehabilitating the two lost functions simultaneously. Provided the floor space allows, a number of patients may be treated together and therefore treatment need not be unnecessarily time consuming. Group therapy has a very beneficial effect. The cheerful, go-ahead patient will encourage his slower companions and competition in progress will result. Several revolutions in quick succession follows rolling from side to side as a natural progression.

Bridging (Fig. 24 and Fig. 5)

The starting position is supine lying with both hips and knees flexed, feet firmly on the floor. This tilts the pelvis forwards, the opposite position to backward rotation of the pelvis which belongs to the extensor spasticity pattern. The affected shoulder is not in internal rotation. The forearms are pronated and pressure on the forearms increases external rotation at the shoulders (working into the anti-spasm pattern). This position ought to have been thoroughly mastered in the ward and it is used over and over again during rehabilitation with various adaptations. It is used at the beginning of the scheme of exercises in the physiotherapy department because the primitive movements of the trunk are rehabilitated first. As soon as 'bridging' (Fig. 5) is achieved actively, *resistance* may be given bilaterally (Fig. 24), or one side at a time to initiate pelvic rotation. The limbs are in the anti-spasm pattern so as much *resistance* as the patient can tolerate may be given. As soon as the patient has learnt to lift his pelvis and hold the position, and to lift alternate hips and hold the positions, he may be taught to rotate his trunk to the affected side by pushing down on the sound leg and to rotate to the sound side by pushing down on the affected leg. Another progression is made when he learns to 'bridge' and then lift one foot off the floor, flexing hip and knee, without lowering his hips. All these exercises do invaluable groundwork in preparation for the normal use of the legs in everyday living. The physiotherapist will plan her own programme of exercise but all physiotherapists will use the basic starting positions, remembering the importance of working into movement patterns which reverse the patterns of tonic contraction. For example (Fig. 11), side lying with one-arm support may be practised while the patient holds the starting position for 'bridging'. The physiotherapist will at first hold the affected leg in position and hold the affected arm well forward with the forearm placed firmly on the floor. The patient is now ready to reach forward and to the left (as he did when he reached for his locker) and lift himself upwards and sideways as he rolls round to prop on his left elbow. If he did not achieve this position satisfactorily in the ward, the physiotherapist may find it necessary to support his leg position with her body as she kneels beside him, and to hold his left forearm firmly in position with her left hand while she assists his forward rotation with a cross grasp, her right hand clasping his right hand. He balances on the left forearm, the elbow directly below the shoulder, and in achieving this exercise he is stimulating the postural reflex in three ways: (a) by moving the position of his head in space; (b) by cross facilitation, or working through the sound side of the body to the affected side; (c) by approximation, weight being transferred from the elbow through the shoulder.

Again it can be seen how closely ward routine and physiotherapy routine ought to be linked, each complementing the other and offering continuity of treatment by way of repetition, identical handling, and a reasoned and hopeful approach which defeats the problems involved and therefore shows a steady and satisfactory progress.

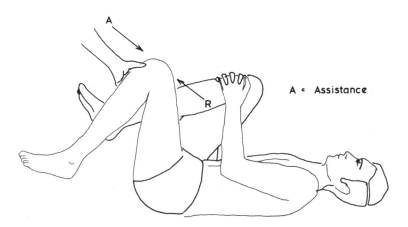

FIG. 25: Re-educating hip flexion.

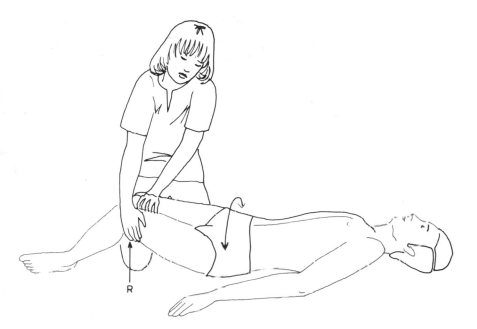

FIG. 26 : Back lying hip rotation.

Hip flexion (Fig. 25)

With starting position as for bridging, the patient flexes his sound leg and holds it in position as shown in Fig. 25. This serves two purposes. Flexion of the sound leg tilts the pelvis still further and makes active holding of the affected leg easier. The patient's hand clasp position holds the humerus away from the forbidden internal rotation pattern at the shoulder. Flexion of the affected hip is then taught, working through the stages of *assisted* movement, *holding* with the foot raised off the floor, and *resisted* movement. For resting periods the legs return to the crook position—never to extension of hips, knees and ankles. Where loss of sensory discrimination is marked in the foot, this exercise may be done with a foot and ankle pressure splint in position. The splint will also stimulate dorsiflexion of the toes and ankle by pressure on the plantar aspect of the toes and it is therefore useful where spasm is marked.

Hip rotation (Fig. 26)

Hip rotation, as shown in Fig. 26, should be taught, bearing in mind that this movement is initiated from the pelvis and hip, and recovery of motor function is from proximal to distal. Trunk—hip patterns must be used in the initial scheme of exercise. Again, with the starting position as for bridging, the patient is suitably placed to counteract extensor spasticity. The hands ought not to be close in to the body. With correct positioning, resistance may be given without

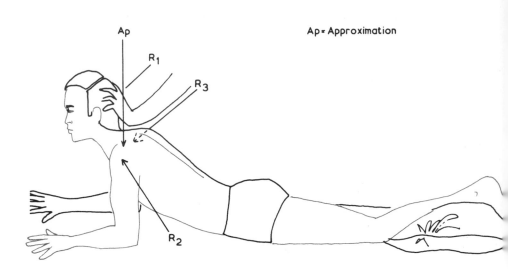

Ap = Approximation

FIG. 27: Prone lying with elbow support.

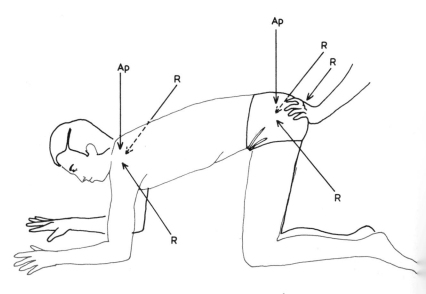

FIG. 28: Kneeling with elbow support.

hips s/b
over knees

building up spasm. The shoulders must both be kept firmly on the floor, the rotation which takes place between the shoulders and the pelvis inhibiting extensor spasticity. This exercise is an important component of rolling when rolling is initiated from the hip and pelvis, and therefore of primary importance in the re-education of the lost postural reflex mechanism and the return of controlled and deliberate movement. Gross movements return first.

The pattern the physiotherapist's treatment follows should now be understood by all members of the rehabilitation team. Re-establishment of postural reflexes leads to re-establishment of controlled and deliberate movement, gross movements (or primary trunk movements) returning first, followed by movements from proximal to distal, i.e., hip to knec to foot, or shoulder to elbow to hand.

Prone lying with elbow support (Fig. 27)

Prone lying follows hip rotation as a fairly easy progression, the roll over to the prone position being initiated by hip rotation and where necessary the physiothcrapist is ready to give assistancc. The patient lies supported on his forearms as in Fig. 27, and the forearm support is the position he should have been using in the ward to lean on a table. The forearms are parallel, *pointing straight forward,* so as to prevent internal rotation of the humerus. In prone lying the elbows must be directly below the shoulders, *approximation from elbow to shoulder* again being the important factor and this is reinforced when the physiothcrapist gives manual pressure downward through the shoulder. The wrist and fingers must be extended with the fingers and *thumb abducted. Resistance* offered laterally to the affected shoulder will correct the starting position each time the patient sags over the sound side. Care must be taken to see that the patient maintains the starting position correctly for all prone lying exercises as in Fig. 27. The affected leg must be placed in slight flexion.

It may take several days to establish each starting position, in particular prone lying with elbow support usually takes some days of training to establish holding of the affected arm in the correct position, but it must be done. Exercise performed in a bad position can do more harm than good. As soon as the position is established, with the weight of the trunk firmly and squarely supported on his forearms, the patient is taught to extend his head against *resistance,* he is taught to transfer his weight from side to side over the forearms keeping his affected hand in the correct position, wrist extended, fingers and thumb abducted, and he is taught to hold the starting position while *resistance* is given laterally to the sound shoulder and laterally to the affected shoulder.

In prone lying, flexion of the affected knee is taught by *active assisted* movement leading on to *active* movement and later to *resisted* movement. *Holding* with no support in various degrees of flexion is a later progression.

Kneeling with elbow support

Prone lying with elbow support (or more correctly forearm support) as in Fig. 27, leads next to kneeling with elbow support as in Fig. 28. The forearm support

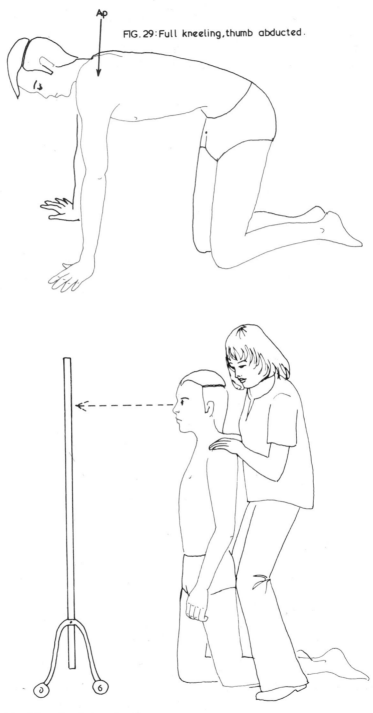

Ap

FIG. 29: Full kneeling, thumb abducted.

FIG. 30: Stand kneeling (using mirror).

has been termed elbow support to emphasise the approximation that takes place between elbow and shoulder. Initially this progression is achieved quite simply if the physiotherapist stands astride her patient, bends forwards to place her hands firmly round his iliac crests and lifts him upwards and backwards into the kneeling position. As far as he is able he assists in the movement and draws his forearms backwards to achieve as nearly as possible 90 degrees of flexion at his shoulders, hips and knees. He is then *stabilised* in this position, that is, he is taught to balance, holding the position firmly against *resistance* offered from various points. *Lateral stabilising* must not be forgotten and the exercise must not develop into a battle of strength. *Resistance* is offered firmly and gently and built up slowly and withdrawn slowly. When the patient maintains a steady position against reasonable *resistance* from any direction he is said to be *stabilised*. Once again it is necessary for the physiotherapist to make sure that his affected hand and forearm are correctly positioned so that firm *resistance* will not lead to build up of spasm in the affected arm. Transference of weight from side to side over alternate forearms is again practised and this is followed by transference of weight from side to side over both limbs. Approximation by manual pressure from hip to knee must not be forgotten.

Full kneeling, thumb abducted (Fig. 29)

Our patient has now been weight bearing from shoulder to elbow and from hip to knee but the arm has not been fully in the anti-spasm pattern. To achieve this he must get up onto his hands in *full kneeling* as shown in Fig. 29. It may be necessary for the physiotherapist to support the affected arm, holding the hand flat on the floor (fingers and thumb abducted) and the elbow in extension. The physiotherapist then removes the support she has given to her patient's hand and transfers *resistance* to the back of his head with his neck held in extension. This equalises the muscle tone in the arm (provided the arm is in the anti-spasm pattern) and allows triceps to contract. Thus, with *resistance* given at this key point of spasm control, triceps contracts and support may be withdrawn from the elbow. The patient is now weight bearing from shoulder to hand. Once again he is *stabilised* in this position. Exercises should be done in front of a mirror. This encourages him to hold his head up, keeping his neck in extension, and sensory input is stimulated by vision. Where there is marked cortical sensory impairment with *agnosia,* or lack of recognition of the affected limbs, mirror work is essential.

He is now ready to begin exercises in crawling.

He is taught to rock backwards and forwards slowly. With *resistance* to backward rocking he pushes on his arms using elbow extension. Lateral rocking is also taught. It should be a slow movement and he is encouraged to hold his weight well over the affected side, balancing on the arm and leg. In a later progression he will weight bear in this position while he lifts the sound limbs off the floor. Modified P.N.F. crawling exercises may be used but the anti-spasm positions of the affected limbs must be maintained and therefore the danger of building up spasm through *irradiation* eliminated. Also the physiotherapist has

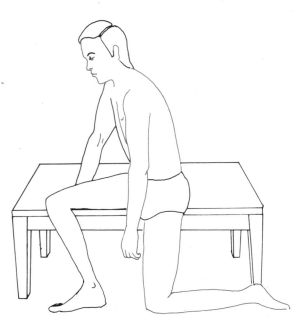

(a)

FIG. 31 (a & b): Getting up from the
floor on to stool.

(b)

to remember that crawling forward is a flexor dominant pattern of movement while crawling backward is an extensor dominant pattern. Therefore, crawling backward is a useful exercise to promote elbow extension, while crawling forward promotes hip and knee flexion. This suggests that the physiotherapist ought to crawl behind the patient so that she may give *resistance* to the front of his thighs while he crawls forwards, and *resistance* to his buttocks while he crawls backwards. In patients where strong extensor spasm of the leg has been allowed to develop, exercise may be done with the foot in a pressure splint.

Stand kneeling (Fig. 30)

To achieve this position the physiotherapist may again stand astride her patient's legs and this time she places her hands firmly on the anterior aspect of his shoulders and assists him into the upright position. Hip extension may give difficulty at first and she may find it necessary to support him with her knees as in Fig. 30. When the position is *stabilised* she kneels on his affected side and gives support through the left hand and arm as shown in Fig. 14a—arm in outward rotation, elbow extended, thumb abducted and weight transferred from the shoulder to the heel of the hand. Weight transference from side to side is practised next, again moving as far as possible over the affected side. Next, knee walking is taught. This exercise must be carefully and thoroughly mastered. It is most important because in this position the patient is using his hip in the correct pattern for normal walking without allowing it to move into the extensor pattern. He is in fact performing formal balanced walking with weight transferrence over the affected side. (Continue to note arm position Fig. 14a).

The whole scheme of exercises must be repeated over and over again, care being taken to maintain correct starting positions at all times and to establish routines which maintain and work into the anti-spasm patterns. The scheme of exercises must only progress within the patient's capability: several days spent in establishing a correct starting position or a minor progression will save time later and give a reasonable hope of full recovery. It is essential that the patient enjoys treatment and is encouraged by it, not defeated by it. The all important arm routine, with and without the use of the pressure splint, may be inserted in the middle of a treatment session. The twenty minute period with the arm in the splint (Fig. 19) makes a welcome rest period and this is followed immediately by the arm and shoulder exercises. If no hand and wrist splint is available for use in re-education of elbow extension (Fig. 22) the half arm splint is removed and re-applied so that it only includes the hand and wrist. The elbow is then flexed, taking the hand towards the forehead, and *resistance* is given to elbow extension. Note the starting position with the arm at shoulder level. All shoulder and arm exercises are again repeated with the splint removed.

Getting up from the floor onto a stool (Fig. 31 a,b)

If correct training procedures have been followed it is very quickly found that getting up from the floor does not present any problem. A solid wooden stool of

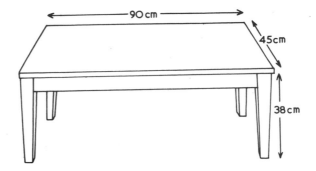

FIG.32 : Suitable stool for training sitting balance.

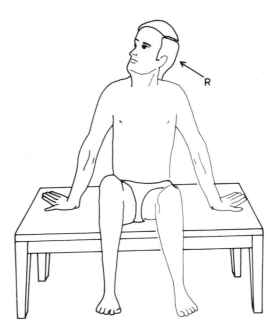

FIG. 33 : Sitting , neck extension against lateral resistance ,
weight -bearing through affected limbs.

the size suggested in Fig. 32 is ideal. From the stand kneeling position alongside the stool, the patient places his sound hand firmly on the stool, lifts his sound leg forward to place the foot firmly on the ground, and leaning on the hand and foot he raises his body until his buttocks are just above the level of the stool and he pivots round into a sitting position. If in any doubt about the correct procedure involved, Fig. 31 (a,b) is self-explanatory.

Use of the stool in rehabilitation

The stool is used to stabilise the patient in sitting and for sitting exercises in CROSS FACILITATION.

Stabilising in sitting

Balance has been established, or training has begun towards this end, in crawling and kneeling, and it must be thoroughly established in sitting before walking re-education begins. Sitting on the stool where the patient has no backrest to depend on is the first step towards full re-establishment of sitting balance. The patient is taught to sit with both arms extended in outward rotation (or external rotation), thumbs and fingers in abduction as in Fig. 33. *Resistance* given laterally on the affected side with the head in extension will assist in maintaining weight over the affected arm and, providing the arm is fully in the anti-spasm pattern, equalising muscle tone so that the triceps will contract and the arm will hold the position and support the body. Next, if the operator places both her hands on her patient's shoulders and applies sudden pressure downwards, postural reflexes are further stimulated. This exercise is most effective if the patient tilts his head backwards so that *resistance* is applied by contact between the back of his head and the operator's body. His spine is then perpendicular in extension and sudden short sharp pressure thrusts are given to both shoulders. This is followed by a longer, firm pressure downwards while he is told to 'hold' and the direction of *resistance* from the operator's hands changes (without moving the hands) to make him 'hold' against rotation of the shoulders. He must learn to 'hold' rigidly so that no rotation takes place. If his hands are kept correctly positioned (Fig. 33) there will be no build up of spasm in the affected arm and in sitting the leg is maintained in the anti-spasm pattern.

As soon as sitting balance has been established, resistance is once more given to the trunk in all directions, gently and firmly at first, building up into strong resistance but, again, this must not develop into a battle between the operator and the patient and again care must be taken to maintain the arm in the anti-spasm pattern. *Lateral stabilising* in hemiplegia is most important. It is a help if each exercise in lateral stabilising is preceded by a short session of downward pressure from the operator's hands through the patient's shoulders. Lateral *resistance* follows, and training sessions must continue until lateral balance is firmly established.

Exercises in cross facilitation

Exercises in cross facilitation are readily carried out when the patient is able to sit on the stool with sitting balance firmly established. Cross facilitation is comprised of exercises which are performed diagonally across the body where the sound side is used to facilitate the weak side by improving postural reflexes and giving sensory stimulation which together improve awareness of the affected side and promote a return to normality. *Irradiation,* or an overflow of muscle activity from the strong side of the body to the weak side, also assists in cross facilitation and, once again, spasm is not produced in the affected arm and leg when they are correctly positioned. Irradiation must not be allowed to take place where it is not possible to maintain both affected limbs fully in the anti-spasm patterns and a build up of spasm can be seen to take place. An example of a useful exercise in cross facilitation is shown in Fig. 34. The patient sits on the stool with his affected arm in external rotation, thumb and fingers abducted, and, leading with the sound hand and following the movement with his eyes, he rotates his body over the affected arm. A cup of tea or coffee correctly positioned on the affected side stimulates exercise performance. It is important that where possible the reasoning behind each exercise should be explained to the patient. This will also stimulate his efforts and understanding will give complete co-operation. Communication must be a two-way process, between members of the team and between the team and the patient.

Rotation of the body over the affected arm (Fig. 34) quite clearly demonstrates the use of three of the basic principles used in rehabilitation in hemiplegia:

1. Working into the *anti-spasm pattern* (the arm is correctly positioned) which balances muscle tone and allows the weak elbow extensors to contract.

2. Giving *approximation,* by weight bearing from shoulder to hand, which stimulates the proprioceptors supplying the joint structures and therefore stimulates postural reflexes.

3. Using *cross facilitation* where the sound side of the body rotates over the affected side and the sound side promotes normal reactions and body awareness in the affected side.

The reasoning behind many of the exercises can be explained to most patients in very simple terms. The aim ought to be for a return to home and normal living as soon as possible, and the more the patient understands about his physical condition and the necessary steps that must be taken to re-establish normal function, the more readily and intelligently he will be prepared to continue his own rehabilitation in his home surroundings when the time comes.

With sitting balance established on the stool, again the physiotherapist will work out her own scheme of exercises to be done in this position, but she will always work into the anti-spasm patterns and any other member of the team who sits in on a treatment session will by now fully understand her aims and the methods she uses to achieve these aims.

Fig. 35 shows a useful leg exercise which may be used to strengthen the knee flexors *provided the arm is held in the anti-spasm pattern.* Again it must be stressed that *irradiation* or *overflow* of activity must not be allowed to activate

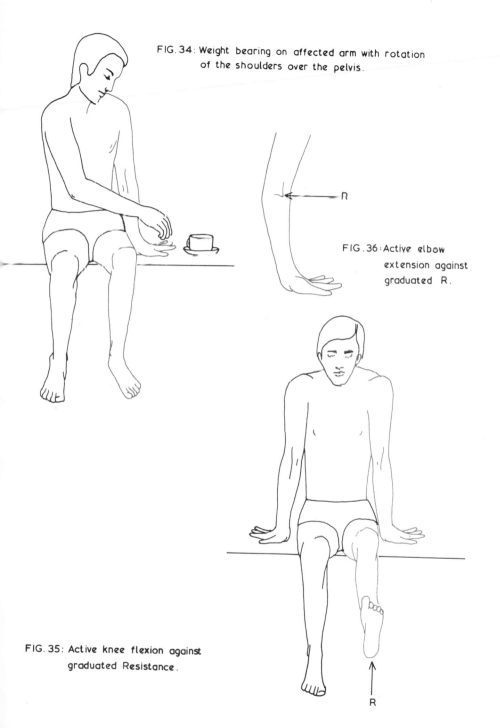

FIG. 34: Weight bearing on affected arm with rotation of the shoulders over the pelvis.

FIG. 36: Active elbow extension against graduated R.

FIG. 35: Active knee flexion against graduated Resistance.

the patterns of the hypertonic muscles. *We are reversing the patterns of tonic contraction.* At no time must this basic aim of treatment be forgotten and it cannot be emphasised too often. The starting position for the exercise is as shown in the diagram with the knee in slight flexion. Graduated *resistance* is given by the physiotherapist at first, and later by the use of spring or pulley. The same exercise may be done to advantage on the sound leg, this time from full extension of the knee to 90° of flexion using strong *resisistance* provided special care is taken to ensure that *irradiation* does not activate the hypertonic muscles in the affected arm—in other words, the arm *must* be held in the anti-spasm pattern. Correctly performed, this exercise will use the sound leg to assist in stabilising in sitting by encouraging the patient to lean forward. Weight-bearing on both arms which are held in the anti-spasm pattern will prevent tonic flexor spasm in the affected arm, will promote postural reflexes, and will initiate active contraction of the weak antagonists on the affected side, e.g. triceps and hamstrings.

Maximal resistance is the greatest amount of resistance which can be applied without defeating the purpose of the exercise. Therefore, in hemiplegia, maximal resistance is *the greatest amount of resistance which can be applied without producing activity in the hypertonic muscles.* From now on, maximal resistance will be referred to as R in the text. Also, the physiotherapist will be referred to as the operator because it will often be necessary for those who are not physiotherapists, e.g. nurses, occupational therapists, district nurses or the patient's family, to assist in rehabilitation. Having reached the stage of firm sitting balance it is time, if possible, to have a member of the patient's family sit in on a few treatment sessions. Re-education will have to continue after he goes home if he is to be given a reasonable hope of returning to full and normal living. The family member as well as the patient will be educated in what must be done.

Fig. 36 shows a valuable arm exercise. The patient remains sitting on the stool with both arms in the anti-spasm pattern (Fig. 33) and alternate active flexion and extension of the affected elbow is practised. Graduated R to extension may be given (Fig. 36). In this way the patient learns to support himself on his affected arm to perform various activities with his sound hand in *cross facilitation.* Now we begin to move into the field of occupational therapy (O.T.) and where there is an occupational therapist in the team she will take over. *But* the physiotherapist must continue; the two fields must integrate; standing up from sitting and stability in standing must be achieved as soon as possible.

Exercises in the parallel bars

Firstly, the operator must make sure that her patient knows the correct and safe way to approach a chair and sit down on it. The broad based chair with solid forearm supports (Fig. 18a) ought to be used at all times. It must not be a chair that will tip when the patient leans his body weight on one of the armrests. He is taught to walk right up to the chair before he leans forward to place his sound hand firmly on the armrest (Fig. 37). With balance safely established in this position he alters his grip, reaching across with his sound arm to grasp the other armrest and turning slowly towards his sound side he sits down. Drill in this

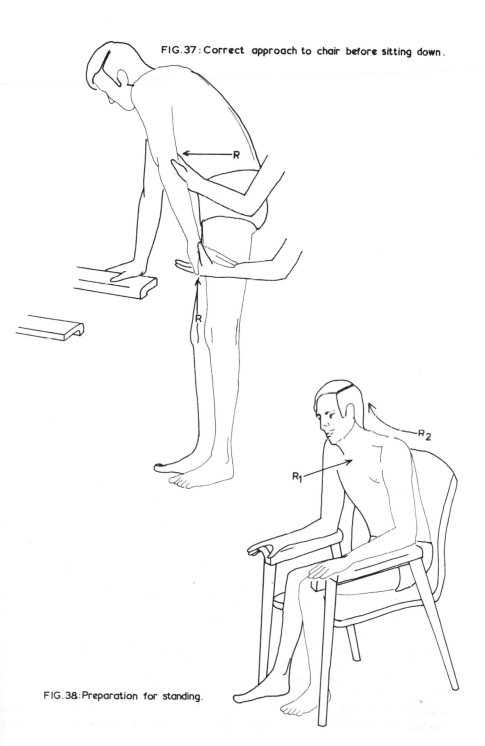

FIG.37 : Correct approach to chair before sitting down.

FIG.38 : Preparation for standing.

movement ought to begin at an early stage. Suitable chairs will be placed at each end of the parallel bars and this safe method of sitting down ought to be automatic, or second nature, when the patient returns home. A correctly positioned mirror should also be placed at one end of the bars. Stability in standing, or standing balance, must now be fully re-established. The patient is seated in the correct chair at the parallel bars with his sound leg placed in front of his affected leg. The first movement towards standing is flexion of the head, head and neck leading, trunk following. This will help control and lead to independent rising. Next the patient is taught to rock forward into the position of trunk flexion against R (Fig. 38, R1) and to sit up again without R. As soon as rocking forward against R1 is firmly established, he is taught to rock against R in both directions. Rocking backward, or spinal extension against R2, promotes extension of the elbows. He is now ready to stand up. Flexion of the head, neck and trunk against R1 is followed by extension of the head, neck and trunk against R2 with traction forwards and upwards while the patient pushes down on his hands. With the hemiplegic patient it may be necessary at first for the operator to teach him to place his sound hand on the arm of his chair and the affected hand is assisted to grasp the bar with the arm well forward in the external rotation of the anti-spasm pattern. The operator then holds the affected hand in position while she gives the necessary R with her other hand. Pulling to standing by using the parallel bars is not advisable; pulling to standing is the least advanced form of rising to standing; pushing to standing by leaning forward and using the arms of the chair ought to be taught.

Having reached an erect position standing in the parallel bars, standing balance is essential to maintain this position. If the patient has achieved standing balance in stand kneeling (Fig. 30) and it has been firmly established, this next advance in his training will not be difficult. Maintaining this erect posture is dependent on postural and righting reflexes and balanced muscle tone, and our whole programme of rehabilitation has been towards this end. Approximation, which stimulates postural reflexes, is applied by manual pressure downward from hips to feet. The operator places her hands on the patient's hips (iliac crests); firm manual contact is necessary; and gives strong pressure in short, sharp thrusts downwards (Fig. 39).

To stimulate postural responses further, R should be given in all directions using head, shoulders and pelvis and rotation must be included. It must be remembered that R given posteriorly gains an extensor response in the legs, and therefore strong R which promotes a strong response will promote the undesired pattern of full extensor spasticity in the affected leg. Again, lateral stabilising for the hemiplegic patient is most important. *When standing balance has been thoroughly established the patient is ready for walking.*

Early walking where a patient is dragged, staggering round a ward or physiotherapy department between two operators, can only lead to a build up of patterns of tonic contraction, muscle imbalance, little or no future chance of reversing the patterns of tonic contraction and a 'victim' who will shortly be condemned to a state of half-living—dependent on the state care of a unit for the disabled, or dependent on members of his family with inevitable frustration and

FIG.39: Standing position for stabilising.

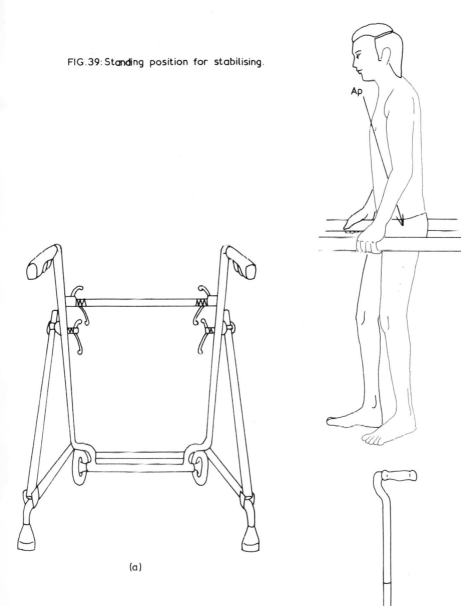

(a)

FIG.40(a&b): Walking aids.

(b)

heartbreak to follow. All through the programme of rehabilitation he must be assessed and reassessed and each step forward must be mastered before the next step is taken. Then, and only then, will he be given a reasonable hope of a return to a full life.

There is also hope for those 'victims' who arrive in hospital, or in the physiotherapy department, some considerable time after the onset of the stroke. The same procedure is followed *but* reversing the patterns of tonic contraction plays a large part in treatment and it must be remembered that even if the patient is on his feet and walking after a fashion, movements are not being initiated from the affected side and it is necessary to go right back to the beginning to train postural reflexes and righting reactions on the affected side. The use of the pressure splint on the arm makes late treatment not only possible but often surprisingly effective.

I hesitate to include walking aids. If it has been possible to follow the rehabilitation programme from the beginning a walking aid ought not to be necessary. If length of stay in hospital does not permit thorough establishment of standing balance, and regrettably it may not, a walking aid must be used. But without full standing balance there are two main problems. Firstly, the lack of postural reactions of the affected leg make for hesitant and unsafe weight transference onto that leg, and secondly, without full re-education of postural reactions and consequent balancing of muscle tone, the affected leg will move readily into the pattern of extensor spasm to make normal walking impossible. The end result is a leg that cannot support the body weight fully and it cannot move forward to take a step without moving as a whole in circumduction with complete lack of localised intrinsic movement. Hence the importance of rehabilitating *lateral stability*.

The Rollator walking aid, as illustrated in Fig. 40a, may be used as a useful adjunct to training for normal walking. With the Rollator held stationary by the operator, the patient is taught to hold his stance with both arms in external rotation at the shoulders, elbows and wrists in extension. The correct arm position is easily obtained at this stage if the handgrips are lowered so that the patient has to lean forward at the hips to grasp them, external rotation occurring at the shoulders automatically when the hands are correctly positioned on the handgrips and the elbows are in full extension. He is then taught to lean on the palms of his hands while he opens and closes his fingers, to mark time, to transfer his weight over the affected arm and leg, to rock from heel to toe and to balance on alternate legs, the other leg being held in flexion at the hip, knee and ankle. Intrinsic movements are essential to normal walking and the patient must have mobility of knee, foot and toes. While he holds this position on the Rollator walking aid he is ready for quadrupedal, or four-footed, walking. In other words, he is again weight-bearing from shoulder to hand, a very necessary step in any rehabilitation programme, particularly where there is loss of sensory discrimination.

The Quadruped walking aid, as illustrated in Fig. 40b, has nothing to do with quadrupedal walking for the patient. It is the stick which has four legs and it is the type of stick most commonly given to hemiplegic patients. Where a stick must be used, it is probably the best of its type *but* the patient will lean on it and his sound leg while he circumducts the affected leg and the affected arm is drawn upwards into the flexor spasm pattern. It is up to the operator to prevent this from happening if circumstances make it necessary to begin walking before lateral stabilising is established. She must walk beside her patient on his affected side, holding his affected arm *as illustrated in Fig. 14a* while she makes sure that he leans towards his affected side. The affected leg must move forward using hip and knee flexion and then it must support the body weight while the sound leg is lifted forward. The affected arm bears weight from shoulder to hand with the arm in the anti-spasm pattern and does not move into the forbidden flexor spasm pattern which would inevitably be activated by *irradiation* or overflow from the effort of lifting the affected leg forward in the correct pattern movement. Then, and only then, will the Quadruped walking aid (or any stick which is used in the sound hand) play a part in restoration of full function, and in particular, in full arm function.

The physiotherapy treatment given for the rehabilitation of the stroke patient has been fairly simply presented so that all members of the rehabilitation team may understand the procedure used and, also, so that where possible patients who return home in the early days to caring families and the help of social services may be helped towards continuing with home rehabilitation with the aim of optimum recovery.

Conclusion

In a book of this length and with this aim, it is neither possible nor desirable to go into too great a depth in any one subject. The physiotherapist knows what she is about and will work out her own programme of rehabilitation, re-establishing *postural reflexes* on the affected side and re-educating *extension of elbow, wrist and fingers* and *flexion of hip, knee and foot* while developing spasm is prevented by using the anti-spasm positions and *working into the anti-spasm patterns.* Spasm is the only serious problem and, as we have shown, it can be eliminated— and must be eliminated—for full rehabilitation when it will finally cancel out because *balance in muscle tone is achieved* and *normal patterns of movement are re-established.*

If any member of the rehabilitation team does not, and cannot, understand this concluding paragraph, let her follow the diagrams with great care and handle her patient accordingly.

Footnote for physiotherapists

Apart from understanding the problem of spasm and the use of anti-spasm patterns, our aim as physiotherapists must be to gain a *response* from an impaired neuromuscular system. To gain a *response* we must make a *demand.* The *demand* is made by (1) *Voluntary effort* from the higher centres of the brain, and or (2) *Sensory stimulation.* A normal *demand* is part voluntary and part sensory. With the stroke patient the *demand* from the higher centres of the brain is missing or impaired and we must step up the *demand* by adding stimuli from the proprioceptors. In other words we must gain a *response* by stepping up sensory stimuli. We are, therefore, largely concerned with facilitating the neuromuscular system by stimulation of the proprioceptors, or sensory nerve-endings which receive stimuli from movement within the tissues, and we are particularly concerned about the affected arm in our stroke victim. If we are depending on sensory stimulation and sensory discrimination is impaired, it is not surprising that we must use all our skill and practical ability to devise ways of getting over this difficulty. The pressure splint is a new and most effective weapon against the barrier of sensory loss. It bombards the proprioceptors into action, or creates a *demand,* and we gain a *response*. It also has the added advantage of holding the limb in the anti-spasm pattern.

Intermittent pressure causes movement within the tissues, and where there is no spasm the Jobst Extremity Pump, which supplies intermittent and controlled pneumatic pressure, gives an ideal answer. But in stroke patients, spasm and the need to maintain the anti-spasm pattern usually calls for a more continuous pressure. I have found that continuous pressure for ten to twenty minutes gains a *response*. Moving the limb in the correct pattern while the splint is in position steps up the *response* that has been gained and makes full rehabilitation possible. The pressure acts on the proprioceptors of muscles, tendons and joints, therefore it acts against the disorder of the normal postural reflex mechanism, helps the sensory disturbance, inhibits the spasm, and allows the initiation of selective movement patterns. Various firms market this orally inflatable pressure splint and, for a number of years, I have found the ReadiSplint, as marketed by Parke-Davis, to be the best of its type. It is, however, not presently available, and in recent months I have found the Jobst-Jet Air Splint, as marketed by Ross & Hilliard, Bellfield Street, Dundee, to be equally good. In orally inflatable splints pressure is controlled by the limited power of the lungs and the warmth of the breath softens and moulds the inner plastic casing to give all over, even pressure. In most cases the half arm splint extends well above the elbow and it must be applied with the arm in the anti-spasm pattern. A very large patient will require a full arm splint.   Perception and proprioception are closely linked together, perception being the power of perceiving by the senses, or the combining of sensations into a recognition of an object, or sensory discrimination, or proprioceptive sense—the sense of muscular position. Many stroke patients have difficulties which show as *agnosia* (difficulty in recognition) or *apraxia* (difficulty in performance) or both. Poor sense of the position of the body in space, or loss of body image, is frequently present. Sensory perception tests will isolate the patient's difficulty which may be related to vision, superficial sensation, or deep sensation, or all three. Tests in *stereognosis,* recognition of objects of different shape and texture held in the hand, must be done without using the eyesight, wherever there is a disturbance of visuo-spatial relationships, stimulation of the proprioceptors must play an important part in rehabilitation.

Therefore, our rehabilitation programme has inevitably been closely concerned with the techniques of Proprioceptive Neuromuscular Facilitation (P.N.F.) which facilitates the neuromuscular machine by stimulating the proprioceptors. The skill of the physiotherapist lies in her ability to use these basic techniques with discretion. The following points must be remembered:

1. *Maximal resistance* for the stroke patient in any exercise is that amount of resistance which will not allow irradiation, or overflow, of muscle activity into the spasm patterns of tonic contraction.

2. *Manual contacts* provide exteroceptive stimulation and should where possible be directional, purposeful and comfortable, using touch to stimulate a response.

3. *Commands* should be simple and dynamic using hearing to stimulate a response.

4. *Normal timing* can only be a goal of rehabilitation, or the end result, as normal timing is the sequence of muscle contraction in the production of functional movement, and the sequence proceeds from distal to proximal. Here we are concerned with re-establishing the postural reflex and proximal to distal development as in the infant. That is, the stroke patient is going through the process of learning the timing that establishes coordinated movements.

5. *Traction and approximation* have an important part to play in our rehabilitation programme. These techniques use proprioceptive stimuli arising in the joint structures. Traction stimulates flexion; approximation stimulates extension. Approximation is used more than traction but traction can be useful, e.g. to stimulate knee flexion.

6. *Stretch stimulus* improves the quality of any contraction but it is not generally used in treatment of the stroke patient. This is because all components of muscle action must be stretched to be effective and this involves the danger of moving into patterns of tonic contraction.

7. *Re-inforcement*, or maximum contraction of strong muscle groups to recruit the activity of weak or inactive muscles by irradiation, or overflow, can only be used with the greatest of care to activate the weak antagonists on the affected side by using the strong side of the body. Unless the physiotherapist is thoroughly experienced, she is far more likely to increase tonic contraction.

8. *Patterns of facilitation* are not generally suitable because of their nature. They are patterns of mass movements which are spiral and diagonal in character and for this reason move into the area of the synergic patterns of tonic contraction. For example, in the arm the flexion-abduction-external rotation pattern (with the elbow in extension) may seem to be the correct anti-spasm pattern to be used in shoulder re-education, but it must not be used in the early days of treatment as a true P.N.F. pattern of mass movement through a full range. Minimal rotation is allowed in the pivot (the shoulder joint, as shown in Fig. 20b), the shoulder joint being used simply as a hinge and flexion-abduction-external rotation applies to the final position of the movement where a few extra degrees of external rotation have been obtained but no internal rotation has been allowed. Used in this way it is an admirable and very necessary exercise, giving shoulder flexion, abduction and external rotation with the scapula rotating, adducting (medial angle) and elevating posteriorly (acromion), and the clavicle rotates and elevates anteriorly away from the sternum. In the beginning stages

the forearm must be held in supination, wrist extended and fingers and thumb extended with the thumb abducted.

As treatment progresses and triceps contracts to give a reasonably strong action (Figs. 29 and 34), the full Flexion-abduction-external rotation arm pattern may be used beginning with minimal resistance to the weak components.

The antagonistic pattern, extension-adduction-internal rotation, *must not be used,* remembering that extension, adduction, internal rotation is the action of latissimus dorsi and leads strongly into the forbidden pattern of tonic contraction and lateral shortening of the trunk muscles.

The mass patterns of P.N.F., being spiral and diagonal, are three-component movements, and, because one of the components is a movement across or away from the mid-line of the body, it is sometimes wrongly assumed that these movements will assist in re-education of postural reflexes and loss of body image, but it must be understood that, because of the ever present need to stay out of the area of the synergic patterns of tonic contraction, in most instances they should not be used as mass movements. Here, the physiotherapist must use her skill to adapt components of movements to suit her aim, keeping at all times away from any movement which will facilitate spasm and seeking only to facilitate those muscle groups which are opposed to the spasm patterns. The patient must be taught to follow all movements that he makes with his eyes, *sight* helping to stimulate a *response.*

There is also a stage in treatment where an understanding of P.N.F. leg patterns can play an important part but they must be modified. Modification is the difficulty because with correct modification the movement ceases to be a correct or true P.N.F. pattern. To give an example: Extension-abduction-internal rotation *with knee flexion* may be used to stimulate down thrust where necessary, *but* the foot and ankle must be held in dorsiflexion by the operator and *resistance* is given against the sole of the foot. The opposite pattern becomes flexion-adduction-*internal* rotation where the starting position is again with the foot held in dorsiflexion by the operator and traction is used to stimulate knee flexion. It will be immediately obvious to exponents of P.N.F. that these are not true pattern movements but they do have an important part to play in full stroke rehabilitation.

Physiotherapy and occupational therapy are now closely associated and ought at this stage to be working hand-in-hand. If there is an occupational therapist in the team she will have much that she can offer towards the patient's rehabilitation, in particular she will lead him towards independence in self-care but the rest of the team are still deeply involved. For example, it is often accepted that it is the occupational therapist who teaches the patient to get in and out of the bath. For this reason the technique used is included in the occupational therapy section. Any member of the team, *particularly the nurse,* ought to handle this problem correctly from the beginning and then it ceases to be a problem.

At some time during their career, most members of the team question the recovery of brain damage in the rehabilitation of the stroke patient. Cells in the damaged area of the brain are killed, and dead cells cannot recover, so what happens? In dealing with the concept of what happens, the following analogy may be found to be useful. It is in no way complete: however, it does lead to a greater understanding of a rather obscure subject:

The brain consists of cells linked by synapsis. These are lines of communication between the cells. This may be likened to a telephone network. The separate cells are the various telephones and the synapsis are the telephone lines. In any system there is the same number of telephones but the network with the best exchanges and the larger number of lines is the more efficient. Also there exist more alternative routes for telephone calls. As the brain synapsis perform the function of the lines, the more synapsis that are in working order the more the calls that get through.

When the brain is 'hit' by a stroke, various cells are killed. In the imaginary telephone network several call boxes and exchanges are damaged. The only way to get round this problem is to use the alternative lines—the important point is that alternative routes do exist. In such a complex network as the human brain there are very many alternative routes. Finding them requires re-education; no area of the network is put out of commission permanently.

With the brain, when the motor nerve tracts, or, in our analogy, the trunk-lines, are 'hit', the areas of the body affected lose communication. The affected muscles, in the absence of orders from the brain, go flaccid. This is followed by spasm and contraction of the stronger muscle groups. This is involuntary and can only be controlled by correct positioning. In the telephone system, the areas that are cut off must not be allowed to fall into disrepair until a trunk-call finally gets through... that is, the prevention of spasm is of first importance so as to ensure that once the alternative routes have been established the muscles are fit to receive orders once more.

The damaged portion of the brain cannot be cured but alternative paths of control by sensory feed-back must be established by re-education. In this instance, as in the case of the telephone network, the telephone is kept ringing until the exchange finds the alternative route round the damaged area and the call gets through.

In other words, in the language of the physiotherapist, when the *demand* from the higher centres of the brain is missing or impaired, it must be stepped up by adding stimuli from the *proprioceptors,* and, with increased *demand,* by repetition of an exercise over and over again, in time the anterior horn (or motor) cell's resistance is broken down, or its threshold lowered. and a *response* is finally gained. The *demand* produces the *response* and there can only be one response, that is, muscular contraction or activation.

Now it will be fully understood why, if it is allowed to, loss of sensory discrimination can pose such a difficult problem in the rehabilitation of the stroke patient. Because a reflex action is an automatic motor response to a sensory stimulus without the brain being immediately involved, e.g. the quick recovery of the balance of the body to prevent falling after a slip, sensory stimulation must play a major part in rehabilitation. Fig. 41 shows a simple reflex arc which consists of three main structures: 1. *A sensory neurone* made up of sensory nerve endings (in our case proprioceptors), the sensory nerve, posterior root ganglion cell and its nerve fibre which passes to the posterior horn

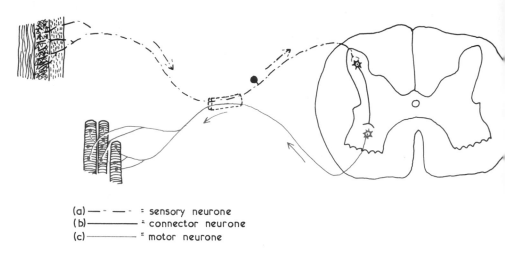

(a) — · — · — = sensory neurone
(b) —————— = connector neurone
(c) —————— = motor neurone

FIG.41: Simple Reflex Arc

of grey matter in the spinal cord;   2. *A connector neurone* made up of nerve cell, dendrites and axon;   3. *A motor neurone* made up of a nerve cell and its dendrites in the anterior horn of grey matter, the axon of this nerve cell and the motor end plates which terminate in muscle.

Pathways or nerve tracts in the spinal cord are *sensory* nerve tracts and *motor* nerve tracts and in our rehabilitation programme we are most concerned with the *sensory* tracts.

The *sensory* nerve tract registers:

1. *Deep sensation* which includes deep pain, *pressure* and the *position of muscle and joint.*

2. *Superficial sensation* such as touch, pain, temperature and pressure. All of these sensations reach the sensory area of the *cerebral cortex*. It is deep sensation which most concerns us.

Thus, in our rehabilitation programme, reflex actions are re-established and carried out very rapidly, and even although the brian is not directly involved messages are transmitted to the cerebrum so that the patient is aware of what is happening. When the sensory nerve tracts of the spinal cord become fully re-educated, which involves reaching the brain, motor nerve tracts are activated and motor response takes over. In the words of our analogy, the telephones have been kept ringing, alternative routes have been established, the muscles have been kept fit to receive orders, and the calls finally get through.

The importance of the sequence of our rehabilitation programme becomes clear. We have: (1) maintained correct positioning to prevent spasm and worked into the anti-spasm patterns to reverse the patterns of tonic contraction; (2) increased pressure on the tissues, deep pressure being used as a means of stimulating the reflex arc and reflex action; (3) stimulated postural reflexes, particularly by using approximation to facilitate proprioceptors. (4) used constant repetition of exercises, particularly in cross facilitation. (5) and finally, we have re-established the postural reflex mechanism and loss of sensory discrimination, and therefore we have balanced muscle tone and re-established normal movement.

Conclusion

In other words, without the use of the pressure splint where necessary to re-establish deep sensation (which includes the position of joint and muscle, or proprioceptive sense) rehabilitation for the stroke patient has had tremendous limitations. In the past the result has frequently been total failure and the residual disability of the hemiplegic arm has been accepted as inevitable. This need no longer be the case. When the importance of the sequence of the rehabilitation programme is studied and understood by the rehabilitation team, this becomes obvious.

4. The Occupational Therapist

Occupational therapy for the hemiplegic patient

Occupational therapy in its truest form means healing by occupation. Much of the activity that takes place in the occupational therapy (O.T.) department may be classed as diversional, and as such it has a therapeutic effect and therefore a part to play in rehabilitation, but nowhere more than in the hemiplegic (or stroke) patient is the aspect of re-establishment of former function by the scientific use of this therapy more necessary. This means that the occupational therapist must be an expert in the handling of stroke patients, she must understand the methods of treatment which facilitate the re-education of the postural reflex mechanism, and she must be always on the alert so that she sets her patient to work into the anti-spasm patterns of movement, rehabilitating the weak muscle groups.

To give a very simple example, and one which ties up easily with what has already been said, for domestic rehabilitation a woman may sit correctly positioned on a stool as already described (Fig. 34) but instead of a cup of tea or coffee she may be given a mixing bowl fastened by suction close to her affected side. She will have the satisfaction of creaming cake mixture with her sound hand while she leans over her affected arm (correctly positioned) and hastens rehabilitation. In the same way a patient may mix a tray of cement, paint a picture, play chess, or do a jigsaw puzzle. These are simple examples. It must be remembered that recovery takes place from proximal to distal and the patient will be at work in the O.T. department long before he has reached the stage of using the affected hand for anything other than holding the anti-spasm pattern while he carries out exercises in cross facilitation. This in itself is of the utmost importance.

Sitting at a treadle loom or machine with the hips and knees in flexion is useful rehabilitation, or, at a later and more advanced stage, exercise may be given standing with the affected side side-on to a lathe with an extended foot plate to encourage dorsi-flexion of the foot with knee flexion while the patient rotates his trunk towards the machine to use his hands in cross facilitation. The raised foot plate prevents full extension of the leg (and thus prevents full movement into the synergic pattern of tonic contraction) and the trunk rotation actively assists in rehabilitation of body image.

These are simple examples. The occupational therapist will use her ingenuity, a quality which is a basic essential in this branch of medical work, and she will adapt and use many and various tasks to assist in the rehabilitation of the hemiplegic patient. To give one more example, sitting at an ankle treadle where the feet are placed side by side, close together and parallel with knees kept together, can be very useful. The agonists, or prime movers, in the foot action are firstly the posterior tibial group of muscles which plantar flex the foot, followed by the anterior tibial muscles which dorsiflex the foot. With the knees in flexion during plantar flexion, complete movement into the anti-spasm pattern is prevented and pressure on the plantar aspect of the toes stimulates dorsiflexion. With dorsiflexion, the anterior tibial muscles are then assisted by the hamstrings in the downward pressure of the heels and the sound leg is used to assist the movement of the affected leg. It can readily be seen what a useful rehabilitation exercise this ankle treadle muscle work gives in the establishment of the intrinsic movements which are essential to normal walking. At a later stage the affected leg may be used without the assistance of the sound leg. Again, bare feet give a boost to sensory discrimination.

Hand machines and foot machines may be (and are) adapted to meet the various needs. When patients are sitting, be it for group therapy round a table or singly, the chair and table must be as carefully selected and positioned as in the ward or the physiotherapy department and the affected arm *must not be allowed to hang in full internal rotation* at the shoulder. Hanging will give traction which is not good, as traction stimulates flexion and it is extension of the elbow which is to be re-educated. Also, internal rotation of the shoulder is the pattern of tonic contraction which has been prevented all through the programme of rehabilitation and which must not be allowed. A sling for the affected arm is not advised. Although it may be applied in such a way as to give pressure on the forearm and stimulation of triceps it encourages internal rotation at the shoulder joint. For rest periods, correct positioning with a suitable chair and table (Fig. 16) is the best solution to the problem of keeping the arm away from the pattern of tonic contraction. For rest periods in group therapy it is equally essential that the table be the right height for the patients to lean on their forearms, both forearms parallel with hands pointing forwards. This keeps out of the pattern of tonic contraction, gives approximation from elbow to shoulder and stimulates elbow extension. If coffee or tea is served, the cup ought to be placed on the affected side so that the patient continues his cross facilitation by rotating over the affected arm to pick up his cup. Correct positioning of the affected arm must always be taken into account when planning the treatment programme.

Group therapy is most important where there is depression and emotional disturbance, and there is frequently a fair degree of emotional disturbance. With speech defect, or difficulty in communication, one of the aims of group therapy is to promote optimism, preventing anxiety and a build up of frustration which leads to complete withdrawal.

Getting in and out of the bath may at first present problems. Properly handled it becomes a simple exercise and purely a repetition of a feat which has already been established. It is exactly the same procedure as getting in and out of bed, and ideally the correct procedure for bathing ought to be established by the nurse in the ward. However, for some peculiar reason, it is sometimes considered to be the duty of the O.T. to establish this procedure and for this reason it is included in this section.

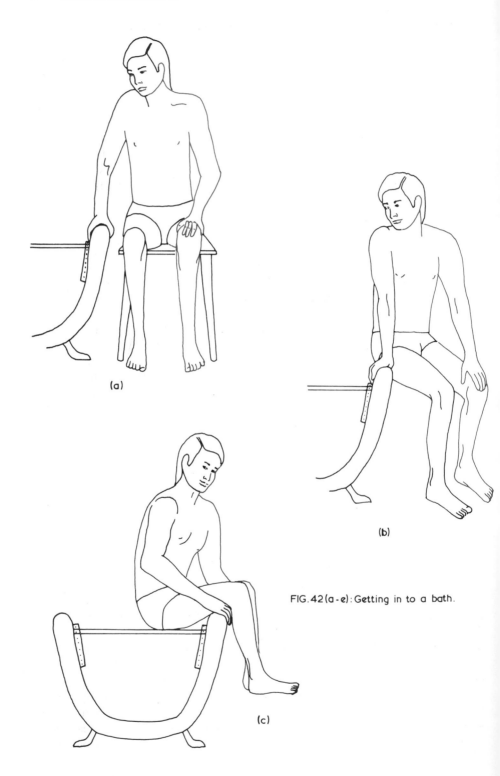

(a)

(b)

(c)

FIG. 42 (a - e): Getting in to a bath.

A non-slip rubber mat is placed in the bottom of the bath and an adjustable bath seat raised to its full height is placed inside the bath. Time spent on a few trial attempts to perfect the following routine using a dry bath with the patient clothed is often time well spent, building up the patient's self-confidence where necessary, allowing full concentration to be given to the actions rather than to the need to wash. If correct handling has been instituted from the beginning there should be no problems.

The patient's chair or stool is correctly positioned beside the bath so that he sits side-on to the bath with his sound side next to the bath (Fig. 42a). If the bath is alongside a wall, so that it is not possible to approach it from either side, it is not necessary to consider where the taps are placed; it is essential to have the patient's sound side correctly positioned.

1. The patient places his sound hand on the side of the bath, stands and pivots a quarter turn to sit down on the edge of the bath (Fig. 42b).

2. He then pushes on his hand and slides his buttocks onto the bath seat (Fig. 42c).

3. Next he transfers his hand to the opposite side of the bath, or ideally to a handrail on the opposite side of the bath or on the wall, and lifts the sound leg into the bath (Fig. 42d).

4. He removes his sound hand from the handrail and assists his affected leg into the bath (Fig. 42e).

The procedure for getting out of the bath is a repetition in reverse. For bathing, a suitable mixing spray for hair washing fastened to the bath taps with the water set at the right temperature will assist his independence, as will a rubber soap sticker fastened to the edge of the bath so that he does not lose the soap. *Cross facilitation* may be brought into use, the soap being placed on his affected side. As his condition improves, the bath seat may be lowered. Eventually he will manage without the aid of the seat.

Dressing may present problems, particularly where the patient has perceptual difficulty, that is, he may not recognise his clothes (*agnosia*), or he may have difficulty in performance (*apraxia*), or in both. This is a disturbance of visuo-spatial relationships. Familiar objects may not be recognised, so the patient may be physically capable of dressing but unable to recognise his clothes or remember how to put them on. Where relationships between vision and space are disturbed, *frustration* must not be allowed to take over or progress will go backwards instead of forwards. He must be given simple tasks that he is able to accomplish and no excessive demands must be made of him. Where there is visual defect, it is related to half of each eye on the stroke side and may demonstrate as hemianopia—blindness of one half of the visual field—or as a sensory disturbance. As rehabilitation continues by careful nursing, by an advancing physiotherapy programme, and by a cheerful and hopeful approach from the occupational therapists, his *apraxic* difficulties will lessen. Where dressing difficulty is due to one-handedness, as it most certainly will be in the early days of treatment, the O.T's will make adjustments to clothing, e.g. velcro fastenings, to give the maximum of independence. Fully established sitting balance is essential.

One of the tasks that has to be achieved in many cases before a patient is

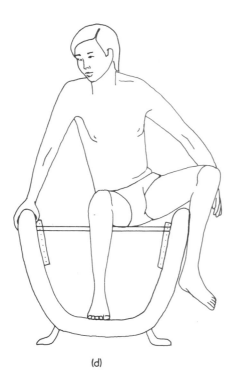

(d)

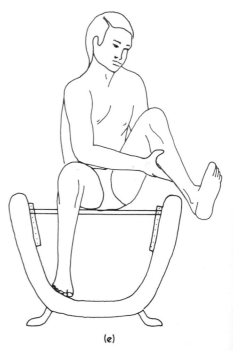

(e)

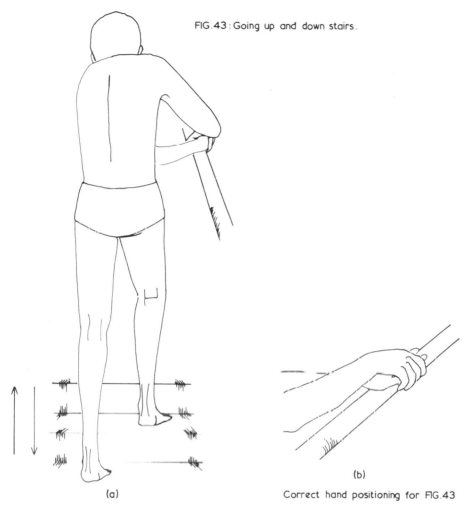

FIG.43 : Going up and down stairs.

(a)

(b)

Correct hand positioning for FIG.43

transferred home is the ability to climb stairs with *absolute safety*. For this, he is taught to take his weight on the affected leg and step up with the sound leg, leaning forward to bring the affected leg up to the same step. Going downstairs he takes his weight on the sound leg and, leaning backward, steps down with the affected leg, followed to the same step by the sound leg. If he is unsure of himself, or unsteady in this exercise, he is taught to go down backwards using his legs in the same order, affected leg first, followed by the sound leg. Take the *good* leg up to *heaven,* take the *bad* leg down to *hell* is a simple way of remembering in which order the legs ought to be used when absolute safety on stairs is the aim. The banister ought to be used where convenient, both hands (if possible) gripping the rail well forward. Where this method is used it does not matter if it is a left-hand or a right-hand rail. When a stick is used it is kept in step with the affected leg. For maximum aid towards full function, normal stair climbing is a useful exercise but it ought not to be used if it will lead to confusion and therefore to lack of safety when the patient goes it alone. That is, if the patient is going home to stairs and therefore safety on his own is of first importance, he ought to be taught the method for coming down backwards and no other. Any other will only lead to confusion. (Fig. 43 a,b).

The occupational therapist will usually make home visits if necessary both before and after the patient is discharged from hospital to assess the home surroundings, to find out if any mechanical aids are necessary, e.g. grab rails in the bathroom, and to make sure that the patient has every chance of achieving full independence.

By stepping up the level of sensory input and working into the anti-spasm patterns, the hospital team is able in many cases to achieve full rehabilitation, and this includes precision movements of the affected hand. The occupational therapists have much to offer towards this final aim.

5. The Speech Therapist

A breakdown in communication

A breakdown in communication between people, and between a man and his normal environment, takes place because of:

1. A motor breakdown which leads to a breakdown in self care and physical contact with others, involving work and home and human relationships.

2. A breakdown in verbal expression.

3. A breakdown in inner control of feelings, emotions, thoughts and desires.

Anything that hinders any or all of these processes leads to a partial or complete breakdown in communication and the patient is no longer in control of his environment. This can be particularly distressing where family, employment and friends are concerned. The patient's whole way of life is threatened and, in total breakdown in communication, he becomes entirely dependent on others. This may, and often does, lead to the patient seeing himself as permanently out of communication and he withdraws still further, cutting himself off completely from all that has made life worth living. He sees himself as useless and worthless and he reacts to this changed image of himself by sinking into deep despair and is often wrongly labelled as bad tempered, difficult and even thoroughly unpleasant.

So far we have seen how the patient can best be helped towards rehabilitation in motor breakdown and, by correct handling and a positive approach to his problems, the inevitable emotional distress has been reduced, but we have not yet touched on *a breakdown in verbal expression.* In no area more than in this field is the team approach to rehabilitation more necessary. No one person can go it alone, and to attempt to do so where there is speech or language disorder is to invite failure. To work as a team we must understand each other, and this means we must understand a little of the language of the speech therapist, or we ourselves will have a breakdown in communication between departments and we shall lose control of our patient's best interest.

The terms that will be used most often are *dysphasia* and *dysarthria* and they must be understood by all members of the rehabilitation team.   1. *Dysphasia* is *a disorder of language* which may include understanding, speaking, reading and writing. It is a disorder of the system of communication through the medium of language and leads to an emotional and social breakdown.

2. *Dysarthria* is *a disorder of speech* which includes difficulty in articulation due to neuromuscular defect of lips, tongue, palate and larynx. It is a disorder of expression involving voice, resonance and articulation.

Dysphasia

The term *dysphasia* is usually used to include all types of central language disorder. In rehabilitation of the dysphasic patient, correct handling from the onset of the stroke is again essential for maximum recovery. Many patients, even although they are not fully conscious, are aware of much that is going on round about them. Even where there is a marked receptive loss, most dysphasics are unexpectedly sensitive to environment and react accordingly. Our team must understand that from the earliest days they must handle the dysphasic patient with the greatest care, expecting him to understand what is going on round his bed, expecting him to understand what is being said. He *must* be given the benefit of any doubt, and at no time must any member of the team talk across his bed as if he was not there. This rule must also apply to the relatives and friends who visit him. We have said 'even if there is a marked receptive loss' but it should be understood that with the majority of hemiplegic dysphasic patients comprehension is good. I have known one hemiplegic dysphasic patient who tore his pyjamas and sheets to shreds from sheer frustration because he was treated like an imbecile when his comprehension was normal. It is important neither to overestimate nor to underestimate the level of comprehension.

Reassurance is of first importance from the onset of the stroke. The patient will be frightened, bewildered and very tired, and he must be told what has happened, where he is and what will be done to help him. It usually does a great deal of harm to try, over and over again, to make the dysphasic patient repeat a word or a sentence. Frustration builds up and the more it builds up the more impossible any improvement in speech becomes.

As spasm must not be allowed to build up in the rehabilitation of normal movement, so frustration must not be allowed to build up in the rehabilitation of normal speech.

Speech rehabilitation is a job that is best left to the expert, but the rest of the team ought to understand how they themselves can best help, particularly by understanding what they must not do.

Early nursing, whether or not there is a central language disorder, is identical, *but* the nurse who does not understand the panic and frustration that accompanies a breakdown in communication through the medium of language can be particularly guilty of unintentionally treating her patient badly. Even where comprehension is lacking, correct positioning and firm handling from the very beginning will give reassurance and lead the patient away from frustration and forwards to a reasonable hope of recovery.

The team must remember that the dysphasic patient shows: 1. Acute anxiety
2. Exaggeration of previous personality traits
3. Surprising fluctuations of performance
Allowance must be made for any, or all, of these symptoms.
The team must remember:
1. To reassure
2. Not to aggravate frustration

3. Not to insist on repetition of single words and phrases
4. Not to isolate, but to provide group therapy
5. Not to lose contact.
There are three types of dysphasia: (1) Executive; (2) Receptive; (3) Mixed.

1. *Executive dysphasia*

Comprehension remains comparatively intact but the patient has word-finding difficulties, or great difficulty in forming words, or a combination of both. There is usually very little speech and what there is is limited to slow laboured words with a tendency to confuse or leave out words. In severe cases there is either complete inability to formulate even isolated sounds; or sounds can be repeated but not words; or single words may be used but sounds are jumbled out of sequence by substituting a wrong letter or by altering the sequence of the letters. This is called 'literal paraphasia'. *Paraphasia* is a form of *aphasia* in which one word is substituted for another. 'Yes' is frequently substituted for 'No'. The *executive dysphasic* almost always demonstrates *dysgraphia* (difficulty in writing) and the disorder is sometimes linked with *praxic* functions (functions concerned with performance) in this case, a tongue and lip *apraxia*. In slight cases speech is slow and deliberate. Where there is marked word-finding difficulty there may be marked *perseveration,* that is, meaningless repetition of an utterance. Reassurance is essential in executive dysphasia. Communication between the rehabilitation team and the patient *must* be maintained at the highest level possible by all team members understanding his home background and his interests so that they can talk to him freely about the things that interest him most. His favourite newspaper or magazine should be produced.

2. *Receptive dysphasia*

Comprehension is missing, that is, the patient does not adequately understand the spoken word. Severe cases show *agnosia* as already described. *Agnosia* is difficulty in recognition, and in relation to speech it means a failure of visual and / or auditory recognition of language. It is usually associated with *hemianopia,* or blindness in half of the field of vision, and proprioceptive loss of the right side (or the dominant side). The rehabilitation team will, in this case, by now fully understand, particularly where there is proprioceptive or sensory loss, how completely treatment must dovetail from all angles. The careful initial handling by the nurse leads to the careful initial training programme in the physiotherapy department, and both must lead to re-established proprioceptive sense if this type of language disorder is to be rehabilitated. Speech may be fluent but incomprehensible, or jargon. In mild cases comprehension of simple conversation is usually present. In receptive dysphasia the speech therapist is frequently concerned with treatment by means of training auditory discrimination, and her place in the rehabilitation team is essential, her skill having a vital part to play.

3. *Mixed executive receptive dysphasia*

This condition can give the most trouble, difficulty in comprehension being added to the symptoms of executive dysphasia giving mixed language disorder.

In all types of dysphasia it is most important for all members of the rehabilitation team to maintain contact with the patient. His family and friends will fill in his background, occupation, interests and hobbies and the team must keep contact, keeping conversation going and where necessary finding alternative means of communication, filling in with gestures, drawing, miming, etc.. A ready rapport will soon be established where mutual understanding and harmony will develop with the reassurance given by correct handling. Experienced, confident caring brings the hopeful optimism on which all treatment depends.

Dysarthria

Dysarthria, difficulty in articulation because of a motor defect, means in the hemiplegic that speech is difficult to follow. It is slow, slurred, and monotonous, but there is no reading problem, therefore there is no language problem. In the language of the speech therapist, the treatment in this case is *unremitting voice and articulation practice.* Exercises are given for the tongue, the lips, in breathing, in using words and phrases, and then, with the encouragement of the speech therapist and the perseverance of the patient, these exercises and phrases are incorporated into speech.

It is up to the nurse to see that everything is done to help the patient towards better articulation. Dentures must fit, he must be able to hear; if a hearing aid is worn it must be in full working order; and his eyesight must be checked. Remember also, because of motor involvement, the dysarthric patient may have difficulty in writing and the speech therapist may help with retraining of motor skill in writing if the hemiplegia is on the preferred side.

When dealing with speech disorders, sentimentality is not helpful; sympathy combined with common sense must be offered so that the patient realises that he is understood and he is going to be helped towards recovery. In this way he will gain the support and reassurance he so urgently needs. Dysphasia may include sensory, visual, auditory and motor defects while dysarthria is a motor defect. If a stroke affects the dominant hemisphere, or the dominant half of the brain, there will be a speech or language disorder. This, therefore, usually applies to right-sided strokes. Most of us have come across the singing dysphasic patient who has marked central language disorder with little or no speech and yet is word perfect when singing a former familiar song. This is thought to be because music, as opposed to speech, is interpreted by the opposite cerebral hemisphere. Music therapy is important. Every possible means of communication must be used to maintain contact with the patient. This obviously includes, in many cases, establishing a non-verbal language in which mime and music have a part to play.

6. Conclusions

'*Wisdom is the principal thing; therefore get wisdom: and with all thy getting get understanding.*'

We set out to discuss treatment for the *complete* stroke but we must inevitably have come to the conclusion that there is much we can do to serve the best interests of all hemiplegic victims at whatever the level of recovery. We must also have reached the conclusion that without skilful and intelligent handling and after-care there is much that can be done to retard or actively prevent possible recovery.

In a book of this length it has only been possible to give the basic principles of rehabilitation in what must surely be one of the most absorbing and fascinating conditions that pass through the hands of the hospital team. Each case is a jigsaw puzzle, every case has certain pieces missing while some cases have extra pieces missing. Find those missing pieces, that is, assess the damage, and rehabilitation becomes comparatively straightforward. Every case is a challenge and every case is a human being who desperately needs help and understanding.

We have also touched on some of the rather obscure and difficult problems which may face our patient. The greatest hurdle in the way of recovery is cortical sensory impairment which gives loss of sensory discrimination, loss of body image and a disturbance of visuo-spatial relationships. Apraxias, which can present enormous problems, probably stem from sensory loss. Agnosia, or difficulty in recognition, can mean that the patient does not recognise the affected side of his body. It may even go as far as *anosognosia* which simply means he does not recognise the disability in the forgotten half of his body, or denies ownership of the affected limbs.

As long as proprioception remains defective we have seen that recovery of normal movement is impossible because of missing sense of joint position and movement. Wherever possible we must begin rehabilitation with correct positioning and rolling from side to side and progress step by step through the infant stages.

All through the rehabilitation programme our aims have been simply stated. Again, we must also have reached the conclusion that in almost every case it is essential to *step up the level of sensory input.* Ways and means of increasing sensory input must be found. New hope is offered to the residual disability of the hemiplegic arm by using the pressure splint to step up sensory input and to work into the anti-spasm patterns. There need be no residual disability. The arm splint must be applied with care, the arm being placed in the complete anti-spasm pattern, and the fingers must not be allowed to extend beyond the area of pressure which, on the air splint, is marked by a red line. Firstly, this is because the end of the splint is open and without pressure on the finger-tips circulation will be constricted and, secondly, for our purpose, pressure on the finger-tips triggers off one of the key points of spasm control.

To generalise is dangerous; no two patients are exactly the same, but to give some idea of recovery time it is necessary to generalise. Starting from the beginning with correct handling, there is usually an initial stage of about two weeks of intensive nursing care with correct bed positions being used at all times. This is followed by correct handling to get in and out of bed, to establish sitting balance and to teach correct positioning with the important arm pattern for sitting at a table. Eight to ten weeks of intensive physiotherapy come next, exercise tolerance being taken into account. This may be followed by a further eighteen months of supervision where convalescent units, out-patient departments and domiciliary services are closely involved. Where correct handling has not been instituted from the beginning, or rehabilitation has been undertaken with lack of knowledge and therefore with adverse effects, recovery time will be considerably longer, if indeed recovery takes place at all, and *residual difficulties will be irreversible*. Where sensory loss is minimal, in the hands of an expert team, the patient's recovery is rapid. Where sensory loss is marked every means possible must be used to step up the level of sensory input. Vision, hearing, cutaneous sensibility and proprioception all play a large part in the rehabilitation programme, and an intelligently planned and careful rehabilitation programme *must* be undertaken.

Treatment in recent years has improved. But it is still possible to come across the hemiplegic patient who was totally neglected in former years and now sits all day in a geriatric unit in the final stages of unyielding deformity where the arm is fixed in the pattern of spasticity and the leg, in spite of previous extensor spasm, has developed fixed flexion contractures of hip and knee. Worse still, the executive dysphasic patient may be left to sit helplessly in this state with a complete breakdown in verbal expression and therefore a complete breakdown in communication with mankind *if* his fellow human beings are ignorant of his communication potential and the reason for his loss of language. And, remembering that his comprehension has remained intact, he is condemned to a life of hopeless frustration and utter loneliness. It is a vicious circle; the more frustration builds up the more impossible any improvement in verbal communication becomes. The future prognosis for hemiplegic victims must not allow this hopeless picture to continue.

New hope will be given, and is being given, to *all* stroke patients where a rehabilitation unit, working as a united team, makes a positive approach to the problems involved. And the only way to make a positive approach is for each unit within the team to understand the methods of treatment used by other departments and the reasoning behind these methods. This leads to complete integration of effort because of complete understanding of the problems involved. Even where total rehabilitation is not possible for underlying medical reasons, there is much that can be salvaged from the disaster and there is a new life to be built.

By establishing efficient hospital rehabilitation teams which offer cheerful, optimistic policy backed by scientific understanding, and which also include family involvement and family education, the hemiplegic victim is given a hopeful outlook and a reasonable prospect of a return to normal living.

Finally, may I again acknowledge the debt I owe to the careful teaching of Professor Norman Dott. Early in my career he gave me a thorough grounding in the complex problems encountered in neurological disability. Under his guidance, the importance of anti-gravity and postural mechanisms, the implication of cortical sensory impairment and the urgent need to step up sensory input where there is loss of proprioception became abundantly clear. It was an honour to be a member of his team.

Glossary

Active movement. Movement where no attempt is made to assist or resist the action.

Active Assisted Movement. Movement where the active action is assisted by an outside force.

Agnosia. Difficulty in recognition.

Agonists. Muscles which contract to produce movement (prime movers) against the weaker antagonists.

Agraphia. Loss of power of writing, from brain disease or injury.

Alexia. Loss of power to read: word blindness.

Anosognosia. Neglect or denial of ownership of the hemiplegic limbs.

Antagonists. Muscles that relax to allow the agonists, or prime movers, to perform a movement.

Aphasia. Inability to express thought in words; loss of the faculty of interchanging thought, without any affection of the intellect or will.

Approximate. To close together with pressure as used when compression is applied through the articulating surfaces of a joint.

Apraxia. A disturbance of visual-spatial relationships, or visual-spatial orientation, which leads to inability to deal effectively with or manipulate objects.

Assessment. Informal but careful observation leading to a decision on the state of the patient and the line of treatment to be followed. Age and general health must be taken into consideration.

Body image. The ability to feel a limb, to appreciate its place in space and its relationship to the body.

Cross facilitation. Working with the sound side of the body across the midline to the affected side to initiate bilateral activity.

Dysarthria. A disorder of speech which includes difficulty in articulation due to motor defect in the muscles of lips, tongue, palate and throat.

Dysphasia. A disorder of language which may, or may not, include difficulty in comprehension. More usually, comprehension remains intact.

Dysgraphia. Difficulty in writing.

Dyslexia. Difficulty in reading.

Euphoria. An exaggerated sense of well being.

Facilitate. To make easy or easier.

Hemianopia. Blindness in one half of the visual field of one or both eyes.

Hypertonic. Excessive, or more than normal, tone.

Irradiation. Muscle activity which takes place where a strong muscle group acts against strong resistance to give an overflow of activity (or irradiation) into other parts of the body.

Muscle tone. A state of slight tension of muscle fibres when not in use which enables them to respond more swiftly to a stimulus.

Paraphasia. A form of aphasia in which one word is substituted for another.

Perseveration. Meaningless repetition of an utterance: tendency to experience difficulty in leaving one thought for another.

Proprioceptor. A sensory nerve-ending receptive of sensory stimuli.

Proprioceptive. (adj.) pertaining to, or made active by, stimuli arising from movement in the tissues.

Proprioceptive sense. The sense of muscular position, or of muscle and joint position.

P.N.F. Proprioceptive Neuromuscular Facilitation. Methods used to facilitate a response from the neuromuscular mechanism through stimulation of the proprioceptors.

Rehabilitate. To restore, to bring back into good condition.

Resistance. Opposition.

Resisted movement. Movement where resistance is given to gain a greater response, or to strengthen the action.

Spasm. A violent involuntary muscular contraction; a state of continuous muscular contraction as opposed to intermittent contraction.

Spatial orientation. Awareness of body position in relation to space.

Stimulus. An action, influence, or agency that produces a response to a living organism.

Synergists. Muscles which contract and relax in conjunction with prime movers crossing more than one joint. N.B. *The synergic pattern of tonic contraction,* therefore, results from hypertonic, or excessive, muscle tone leading to muscle contraction which follows the pattern of the *synergists.*

Index

39
44

Poles
155
135
140
155
~~135~~